STROKE-FREE FOR LIFE

The Complete Guide
to Stroke Prevention
and Treatment

STROKE-FREE FOR LIFE

The Complete Guide
to Stroke Prevention
and Treatment

DAVID WIEBERS, M.D.

A LIVING PLANET BOOK

CLIFF STREET BOOKS
An Imprint of HarperCollins*Publishers*

This book is written as a source of information only. The information contained in this book should by no means be considered a substitute for the advice, decisions, or judgment of the reader's physician or other professional adviser. No decisions regarding diagnosis, prognosis, or treatment should be made on the basis of this book alone.

All efforts have been made to ensure the accuracy of the information contained in this book as of the date published. The author and the publisher expressly disclaim responsibility for any adverse effects arising from the use or application of the information contained herein. No real patient names or specific identifying information has been used in this book. Neither the author nor Mayo Clinic endorses any particular product mentioned in this book.

Grateful acknowledgment for use of illustrations and images by permission of Mayo Foundation.

HarperCollins books may be purchased for educational, business, or sales promotional use. For information please write: Special Markets Department, HarperCollins Publishers, Inc., 10 East 53rd Street, New York, NY 10022.

FIRST EDITION

Printed on acid-free paper

Library of Congress Cataloging-in-Publication Data

Wiebers, David O.
    Stroke-free for life : the complete guide to stroke prevention and treatment / David Wiebers.
        p.   cm.
    Includes index.
    ISBN 0-06-019823-0
    1. Cerebrovascular disease—Popular works.   I. Title.

RC388.5.W466   2001
616.8'1—dc21   00–065688

01   02   03   04   05   FF   10   9   8   7   6   5   4   3   2   1

To my patients

Contents

Acknowledgments

When one reflects on how, over time, a project such as this book ends up being the product of so many others and their influences on one's life, it becomes evident that it is not possible to adequately acknowledge all those who have meaningfully contributed. It is also easy to become overwhelmed with gratitude and filled with joy at having the opportunity to interact with so many generous and wonderful souls.

I am deeply indebted to my friends and colleagues at Mayo Clinic and the Department of Neurology for so many things, including the overall positive, healing, supportive, cooperative spirit which characterizes this wonderful institution; the unparalleled clinical environment that encourages innovation in caring for patients; and the hundreds of individuals involved in the decades of research from the Mayo Stroke Center and other Mayo sources that form the basis for much of the content of this book.

In particular, I express profound gratitude to Dr. Jack Whisnant, my mentor and colleague over the past twenty-five years, who assisted throughout the development of this book and the risk-assessment questionnaire. Jack's selfless guidance and generosity over the years have meant more to me than words can adequately express.

Several other colleagues have also been particularly active in Mayo Stroke Center research and have provided valuable assistance, including Dr. W. Michael O'Fallon and JoRean Sicks, who provided great statistical expertise in the development of the computer program and risk-assessment questionnaire, and Drs. Robert Brown, Irene Meissner, and George Petty, who have also made enormous contributions to Mayo Stroke Center research over many years. Dr. Brown along with Dr. Valery Feigin also coauthored two of our books for physicians, *Handbook of Stroke* and *Cerebrovascular Disease in Clinical Practice,* which helped to provide the basis for some of the scientific content of the current book. Drs. Whisnant, Brown, and Petty along with Dr. Kelly Flemming also provided extensive review and valuable commentary regarding the manuscript.

Drs. James Seward, Teresa Tsang, and Bijoy Khandheria from the Division of Cardiology also provided major contributions regarding theoretical and practical aspects of diagnostic, therapeutic, and preventive strategies and the relationships of cardiac function to stroke and stroke-risk-factor prevention.

I am also very indebted to Sandra Twaites, who provided superb administrative and secretarial assistance; Rita Jones, R.D., and Dr. Donald Hensrud, who provided valuable assistance regarding dietary and nutritional issues; Frank Helminski, Esq., and Jill Smith Beed, Esq., who provided ongoing extensive legal support and guidance; Jane Jacobs, Lisa Copeland, and Suzanne Leaf-Brock, who provided valuable communications assistance; and Drs. Michael Wood, David Larson, Brooks Edwards, John Noseworthy, and Jerry Swanson, who provided considerable support, vision, and guidance throughout this project.

Special thanks to my mother, Helen Wiebers, and to Marge Wise, Steve Ann Chambers, and Rita Jones, R.D., for valuable assistance in providing recipes listed in the appendix of this book.

I cannot say enough about my wonderful publisher, Diane Reverand, and my editor, Matthew Guma. I would also like to thank their colleagues at HarperCollins/Cliff Street including Richard Rhorer, Paul Olsewski, Nathaniel Hawks, Carolyn Hanson, Adam Goldberger, and Charlie Schiff. This dedicated team of people has shown great vision and skill throughout the development and publication of this book, and I am extremely grateful for all their hard work.

I am also enormously grateful to Jennifer Hay for her outstanding work in researching, organizing, and providing content for the manuscript; Josh Horwitz from Living Planet Books for his incredible packaging skills; my talented agent, Gail Ross, for her expert guidance; and my producer, Steve Ann Chambers, without whom this book would not have been possible.

STROKE-FREE FOR LIFE

The Complete Guide
to Stroke Prevention
and Treatment

1

A New Paradigm for Stroke Prevention and Treatment

When I first began my medical training in the 1970s, I was immediately drawn to neurology. What could be more fascinating than decoding the mysteries of the human brain? But many people discouraged me from pursuing this field. The brain was simply too complex, they believed, and the nature of brain diseases too opaque, for doctors to be able to help most people. Better to go into cardiology, I was advised, where life-saving advances were being made in repairing—even transplanting—diseased hearts.

I stuck with neurology because the lure of exploring the uncharted regions of the brain was simply irresistible. The last few decades have been a time of tremendous advancement in our understanding of the way the brain works. The 1990s were rightly dubbed "The decade of the brain," when the advent of new imaging technologies opened a window into the master control room of our consciousness. After centuries of merely guessing how things worked inside our skulls, we now have vivid pictures of neural pathways. We can understand how nerve impulses control various aspects of our physical being, and can even identify the neurological basis for many of our emotions.

In the past few years, breakthroughs in imaging technologies, medications, and surgery—as well as data from population-based epidemiology—have given us dramatic insights into the most prevalent and destructive of brain disorders: stroke. What we've learned flies in the face of many of our most deep-seated assumptions about this dreaded killer and disabler.

For many years, people referred to stroke as "apoplexy," a term derived from a Greek word meaning "to strike down." The word portrays stroke as something sudden, unexpected, unpredictable. An outdated clinical term for stroke, "cerebrovascular accident," carries a similar connotation. These terms no longer apply. In the last few decades—and particularly in the past few years—we have learned what causes and contributes to stroke. We have learned that stroke, though sudden, is neither unexpected nor unpredictable. In fact, in most cases, it represents the end stage of a related disease or condition.

As a researcher who has devoted his career to treating stroke, I find these to be exciting and empowering revelations. If stroke can be predicted, and its causes pinpointed, then it can be prevented. In fact, I believe that up to 80 percent of strokes are preventable. The best news of all is that in the majority of cases, stroke can be prevented through noninvasive changes in lifestyle.

Everyone in health care recognizes that disease prevention saves more money, lives, and suffering than reactive treatment, but up till now, prevention has played only a minor role in stroke medicine. I've written this book to promote a shift toward a new paradigm in stroke treatment: a paradigm of prevention that begins well before old age. Preventing stroke means looking at lifestyle issues and risk factors that begin causing disease in our thirties and forties.

Until we convert our new knowledge about stroke into a coherent prevention program, millions of people are being disabled or killed by a calamity we are failing to avert. The statistics are staggering: Stroke strikes approximately 750,000 Americans every year, killing an estimated 160,000. There are more than 4 million stroke survivors in the United States and almost 30 million direct family members of those survivors. During the course of a lifetime, four out of every five families in the United States will be touched by stroke.

These numbers are tragic, especially since it doesn't have to be this way. We now have the power to prevent most strokes. Prevention is not a passive process. Rather than fearing stroke as an unexpected and inevitable killer and disabler, we need to face it squarely as a predictable medical condition that can be prevented. Each of us needs to take an active role in shaping our medical destiny—first, by assessing our risk level, and second, by taking important steps toward reducing that risk.

Risk assessment has been an imprecise science. We know that certain conditions have increased stroke risk, but we haven't known to what extent and how various risk factors interacted. That has changed. The culmination of four decades of research at Mayo Clinic—along with studies from other medical centers and those we have collaborated on or conducted around the world—has yielded a more complete picture of the numerous variables that increase stroke risk as well as how those variables interact. Our team at Mayo has recently converted this information into a comprehensive method for predicting who is at risk of stroke.

We wanted to make this new risk-assessment tool available to the general public in book form. Armed with the program outlined in this book, any motivated person can create a personalized prevention program.

THE PREVENTIVE POWER OF LIFESTYLE

The newly fleshed-out portrait of the lifestyle and medical factors that can lead to stroke is a powerful preventive weapon. True, this complex picture indicates that no single simple approach can prevent stroke, but it also shows us that stroke is much more deeply rooted in remediable lifestyle risks than has been previously thought. Each of us can have a profound influence on our medical destiny.

I hope this book will give you all the information and advice you need to add years to your life. Rich years, full of family and friends, work and play. It's really up to you. I see a vital role for such lifestyle factors as diet, exercise, and stress reduction in preventing stroke and the conditions that lead to stroke. As more and more lifestyle factors enter into the risk/prevention equation, your role becomes increasingly central. Only you can control such lifestyle risk factors as diet, alcohol consumption, stress, and smoking cessation. Although you will need to work with your doctor to review the various prevention and treatment options at your disposal, the ultimate decision whether or not to take steps to prevent stroke will rest with you.

I believe lifestyle changes should be viewed on a level playing field with drug therapies and surgical and procedural interventions in approaching stroke prevention. Considering that I work in one of the highest-tech medical centers in the world, you may be surprised that I advise my patients to consider the most natural and least invasive treatments first. This is because decades of experience has taught me to respect the delicately balanced nature of brain chemistry, physiology, and anatomy. Drugs and surgery introduce new risks into the calculus of treating any brain disorder.

Drugs are often a valuable part of stroke treatment, and such drugs as Mevacor and Zocor, for instance, have proven to be highly effective treatments for high cholesterol, which can lead to certain kinds of stroke. Every drug has side effects, and using multiple drugs incurs the risks of dangerous interactions that can be difficult to anticipate for individual patients. It's also true that the frequency and seriousness of side effects are often underrecognized and underreported. If dietary changes can achieve the same goals as cholesterol-lowering drug therapies, why not simply eat differently? The more natural dietary approach yields health benefits that far outweigh merely lowering cholesterol without the potential for serious side effects that drugs carry.

Surgery is another potentially lifesaving option that should be considered only along with a healthy respect for potential complications. Operating on the brain or its blood supply is never without risk and is seldom routine. The brain is simply too complex an organ with too many microscopic components. Beyond its anatomical intricacies, the brain remains a largely inscrutable organ. We still don't understand a lot when it comes to cause and effect, which means that opening the cranium and surgically altering brain tissue can always have unintended consequences.

Again, in cases where lifestyle modifications might achieve the objectives of surgery with less risk, why not try those first? My point isn't to diminish the significance of pharmaceutical and surgical advances in stroke medicine—it's to accentuate the potential impact of noninvasive, low-risk lifestyle changes in reducing or avoiding the need for other treatments.

A good illustration of the power of lifestyle changes was Arnie, a fifty-nine-year-old cattle rancher from South Dakota. He grew up eating meat three or four times a day virtually every day, as well as lots of eggs and dairy as I did. When he came to see me, Arnie's cholesterol was over 300 mg/dL, and he had already had coronary artery bypass surgery. Now he had blockages in both his carotid arteries (the main arteries feeding blood to the brain), which can sometimes lead to stroke or temporary strokelike spells, called TIAs, that may precede and foretell a stroke. He also suffered from frequent angina attacks.

Surgery to clear his carotid arteries was one option we explored, but this approach carries some risk, particularly in someone with frequent angina. We decided to take a less invasive approach first. I put him on an anti-platelet drug to avert any immediate danger of losing blood flow to the brain, and I immediately got him into Mayo's very effective smoking cessation program. Then we devised a low-cholesterol diet plan that included a range of meat substitutes. After testing various brands against each other, he quickly found a menu of substitutes that satisfied his lifelong craving for meat tastes, without the health problems it had created. He and his wife, Helen (who also had a 250+ cholesterol), took a lot of flak from the local cattle ranchers for giving up meat, but the substitutes were so satisfying that they didn't miss the sausages, bacon, and hamburgers that had been staples of their diet. After they saw the change in their cholesterol counts, they never looked back.

Within a year, both Arnie's and Helen's cholesterol levels were around 150 mg/dL, and Arnie's carotid artery blockages actually *regressed* on both sides. He looked younger than he had in years and was markedly more energetic and more alert. His chest pains had disappeared. As he told me the last time we met, "Helen and I are feeling so good, we're going to Europe this fall for the first time. We've been planning this trip for years, but with my health so darn unpredictable, we'd been afraid to leave home."

I've witnessed tremendous advances in neurosurgery during the course of my career. The progression from X rays to CT scans to MRIs and PET scans has given surgeons a huge advantage over their predecessors in locating and repairing blood vessels and various lesions in the brain. Surgical technologies like gamma knife radiosurgery have introduced a degree of precision that was unimaginable twenty years ago.

The skill and precision required in neurosurgery are almost superhuman. Simply put, there is no margin for error. The best surgeons understand this and are very selective about when to operate. Though the following case is an extreme example, it illustrates how important it can be to consider noninvasive, nonsurgical treatments, even in dire circumstances. A fifty-five-year-old cabinetmaker named Howard arrived at the hospital one day in very precarious condition. He was experiencing successive transient ischemic attacks

(TIAs, which are essentially mini-strokes) that immobilized all four of his limbs and partially deprived him of his ability to speak and swallow. When we imaged his head and blood vessels, we found that his basilar artery was virtually blocked by atherosclerosis. The basilar artery feeds blood to many of the vital areas of the brain stem.

Howard's TIA episodes would occur any time he sat or stood up, when the uphill blood flow to his brain couldn't penetrate his blocked basilar artery. These were extremely dramatic episodes that confined him to lying down in bed. In fact, we ended up having to put the head of the bed downward in order to have gravity help the blood flow. We explored several very dramatic types of surgery, including one that would dilate the blockage in his basilar artery. We had only performed this surgery a few times before, as last resorts for patients in dire straits, and the results had been mixed.

This was one of those crises that frays everyone's nerves—most of all the patient's. The surgeon we called in was very wary of operating; various complicating factors would make it extremely risky surgery, and he did not have a good feeling about it. I've come to respect the "sixth sense" of good surgeons, and we counseled Howard against the surgical option. He could easily have panicked and insisted that we take dramatic action. After all, he was becoming totally paralyzed for frightening stretches of time. Instead, he showed great patience and courage—which allowed us to recommend using blood-thinning agents and other more conservative nonsurgical measures, as his body healed itself by creating its own collateral blood supply around the blockages. This required several weeks of bed rest in the hospital as well as trust and tenacity on Howard's part.

We were quite amazed and extremely pleased that eventually he gradually began to be able to sit up, and then stand up, and finally, he had no further episodes. From there, we prescribed major lifestyle changes, including diet, exercise, and stress reduction, which Howard was obviously very motivated to embrace. Although not all cases have such a happy ending, this one illustrates the phenomenal potential our bodies have for self-healing—if we can resist the temptation to throw the most technology at every medical condition.

WHY I WROTE THIS BOOK

As with every doctor, my first experience of "losing a patient" is forever seared in my memory. I wasn't a neurologist yet. I was a first-year medical resident when I was put in charge of a woman with terminal lung cancer. Her name was Ginny, and she was fifty-two years old—I remember because she was the same age as my mother at the time, and the idea of my mother dying that young was unbearable to me. Ginny had smoked two packs of cigarettes a day for thirty years. As I watched her die during the course of the week, I couldn't escape the fact that even if I had been a skilled physician, there was nothing I could do to save her. I visited her several times a day and held her hand and tried to make her comfortable, but she was dying, and all I could do was watch.

What I realized that week, and what I come face to face with continually as I practice medicine, is that no matter how much I learn, and how much medical mystery gives way to medical knowledge, healing is a collaborative process. It's something that happens, when it happens, between individual patients, their doctors, and a variety of other positive forces. I want to give you all the information you need to be an informed and collaborative partner with your doctor. The more information you have, the better equipped you will be to make important decisions regarding your health.

I've written this book because I recognize that my patients' knowledge and motivation to get involved in their own treatment are among the most important factors in their medical outcome. Knowledge and motivation are more important than all the technology available in today's medicine. What matters most is my patients' willingness and ability to get actively involved in their own healing. This is where meaningful prevention and treatment really begin.

I've worked at the center of high-tech medicine throughout my career. As a diagnostician and researcher, I do not hesitate to take full advantage of the technology, medications, and surgical procedures at my disposal. In the end, it's the human factor that so often makes the difference: the ability of doctors and patients to communicate effectively, the judgment of a neurosurgeon or neurologist, a patient's intuitive grasp of what course of treatment will prove most effective for him or her. There are still many unknowns in this field, and each individual case remains a puzzle that requires the collaboration of doctor and patient to sort out. The stronger a partner you become in this process, the better off you'll be.

One of my goals in writing this book is to provide readers with the most comprehensive and up-to-date overview of what works best to prevent and treat stroke. Many of my patients like to do their own research and sometimes have had difficulty finding information about their conditions and how those conditions affect stroke risk. They often have had to read about stroke in one source and about their condition in another.

Beyond the hard data I've gleaned from our research and clinical practice, I'll also be offering you my best judgment—which is sometimes simply my best guess based on available research—about what works best in which situations. What's published in medical journals and gradually integrated into medical practice is the result of years of studies, followed by confirmatory studies. As someone who's been coordinating Mayo's population-based stroke research and a large international study of stroke, I can share with you not only what we know to be true, but also what I suspect to be true. I believe strongly in the benefits of research, but I also believe that the dissemination of medical knowledge is often slower than desirable.

Being informed about recent medical advances is important not only for stroke prevention, but also for stroke treatment. Stroke, as I've said, is usually the end stage of an underlying disease or condition. Depending on where you are in the disease process, preventive efforts may come too late. There are some risk factors and conditions over which we still have little or no control. The good news is that there have been tremendous leaps in stroke treatment in the past decade. The growing availability of such imaging technology as computed tomography and magnetic resonance imaging has greatly improved diagnosis. And the advent of thrombolytic drug therapy has given us the first proven acute stroke treatment in the hours immediately following a "brain attack." These drugs can make the difference between life and death or livelihood and disability for many people. To take full advantage of the latest advancements in stroke treatment, you need to know where to go for help—and when to seek it. I've dedicated the latter part of this book to the need-to-know information about how and where to find the best stroke treatment and the most up-to-date stroke medicine centers.

HOW TO USE THIS BOOK

This book is jam-packed with information and is not meant to be read cover to cover. It is designed to provide you with the information you need, in a usable format, to reduce your own risk of stroke. I've included information not only about such common stroke risk factors and causes as hypertension and diabetes, but also about those that apply to smaller numbers of people—sickle-cell anemia and cardiomyopathy, for example. As a result, not all the information will be relevant to you—but you will find the information about your particular condition or conditions. The book is organized so that you can read about what you need to know, and skip over what you don't. It provides you with the information you need:

1. to educate yourself about stroke
2. to assess your risk of stroke
3. to take the steps you can to prevent a stroke from occurring
4. to deal with a stroke emergency and its aftermath should you or a loved one be stricken.

The first part of the book, chapters 2 and 3, is designed to help you assess your risk of stroke. I briefly explain stroke, show you how to assess your own risk, then detail the various risk factors that are relevant to you personally. Though you should be able to complete the risk assessment yourself, you'll want to work closely with your doctor to tailor your prevention program, particularly if your profile turns up medium-to-high risk.

The next section, chapters 4 and 5, is all about stroke prevention. I present an overview of the various tools we have on hand to reduce stroke risk, a risk-factor-by-risk-factor prescription for preventing stroke (cross-referenced from your risk assessment quiz, so that you can read only about those that apply to you), and lifestyle recommendations for reducing stroke risk and keeping stroke risk low long-term.

The next part, chapters 6 to 8, is designed to prepare you to cope with a stroke emergency and its aftermath. I give you a need-to-know list of stroke warning signs and potentially lifesaving advice about where to go for treatment, then outline the various treatments available for stroke, beginning with emergency, or acute, treatment and continuing through rehabilitation. This part concludes with a look forward at the near future of stroke prevention and treatment (chapter 8).

The last section of the book, chapter 9, is a hands-on-guide to surviving stroke, from dealing with your insurance company to getting the most out of your medical team, designed to answer many of the questions you or your family might face or be facing in the future. I've also included valuable resources in appendices at the back of the book.

Throughout *Stroke-Free for Life,* I will suggest ways you can work with your doctor to achieve the best results in prevention and treatment. The patient-doctor relationship has come under a lot of pressure recently because of managed care—which is why it's so important for you, the patient, to take the initiative in becoming an informed and active partner in preventing or treating your stroke.

Stroke-Free for Life will educate you about stroke, help you identify your risks, and empower you to take action to prevent this killer and disabler. I also hope that it will change your thinking about stroke. No longer an unexpected event over which we have no control, stroke is something that we can prevent if we put aside our fears.

When it comes to serious illnesses, like cancer or heart disease or stroke, many of us go through life with blinders on. We can feel helpless, and those feelings of powerlessness can lead to fatalism. When our number's up, it's up.

So many of my patients, working with the support of their spouses and extended families, have been able to take charge of their health and grant themselves decades of life that would otherwise have been lost. And I'm not just talking about physical and mental vigor. I've watched these patients enjoy a peace of mind born of knowledge and action that is as precious as life itself.

I've written this book to help you retain control of your life. If you're reading it, you've already taken the first steps away from fear and fatalism . . . away from disability and death . . . toward health and life.

2

The Anatomy of a Brain Attack: The ABCs of Stroke

Tax time was the busiest, most stressful time of the year for Jack. The fifty-five-year-old accountant put in long hours at the office and paid less attention than usual to his health, living on fast food and cigarettes and forgetting to take his high blood pressure medication. When he noticed a numbness in his left arm, leg, and face, he chalked it up to overwork. The numbness came on suddenly and lasted only ten minutes. He thought it was the result of lack of sleep or sitting in one place too long, so he didn't give it a second thought. Two days later, the numbness returned with a vengeance. This time, his left side was entirely paralyzed.

Marie was working in her garden when her head began to throb. This was no typical headache. It felt as if she was being hit over the head with a hammer. She went in the house to lie down, thinking that might make her feel better. It didn't. In fact, the back of her neck began to feel stiff as well. By the time her husband came home from work, she was unconscious.

Mike was enjoying retirement. He kept busy with travel and volunteer work. One day when he was working at the local food bank, he felt a sudden numbness on the right side of his face, his vision became blurry, and he became disoriented. When another volunteer approached him to ask what was wrong, he couldn't understand the question. And when he tried to respond, the words didn't come out right.

These are the faces of stroke: people from all walks of life, all races, all ages, both sexes. They could be your neighbors, coworkers, friends, or family members. You could be next—and that thought can be frightening.

In twenty-five years of medical practice, I've discovered that patients fear stroke more than any other illness, including cancer. In fact, medical surveys reveal that people are more fearful of being disabled by stroke than of death itself. They've seen how ruthlessly stroke can disable people's minds and bodies, robbing them of speech and cognition, of expression and movement, of control over their lives. They've watched as entire families have been devastated by this seemingly sudden medical event. And they've worried that the same thing could happen to them or to someone they love.

Fear is a double-edged force. It can either paralyze us in the face of danger, or it can motivate us to act to prevent catastrophe. Many patients who have come to me with prestroke symptoms have been motivated by their fear of impending stroke to turn around their medical conditions. I wish some of my other patients had developed a healthy respect for the destructive power of stroke before it affected them.

The facts about stroke are indeed frightening:

- Stroke is the third leading cause of death and the leading cause of disability in the United States.
- Ischemic stroke (the most common type of stroke, which I describe later in this chapter) has a 20 percent mortality rate in the first thirty days. Survival is about 65 percent at one year and 50 percent at five years.
- Between 60 and 70 percent of ischemic stroke survivors have some disability immediately after the stroke, 40 percent at six months, and 30 percent at one year.
- Subarachnoid hemorrhage (one of two types of hemorrhagic stroke) has a 40 percent mortality at thirty days. About half of those who survive are disabled. Statistics for intracerebral hemorrhage (the other major type) are similar.

I hope that grasping the consequences of stroke will have a cautionary impact on your thinking and behavior. Some of stroke's effects resolve on their own and others can be reduced or eliminated through rehabilitation. But regardless of the degree of recovery, a brain attack is a traumatic medical and emotional crisis that we should all seek to avoid if at all possible. And in most cases, stroke can be avoided. The best defense against stroke is to understand what causes a brain attack, assess your individual risk factors, and take steps to reduce those risks.

THE EFFECTS OF STROKE

Part of why strokes are so frightening is that their effects are so wide-ranging. The middle-aged woman experiencing a sudden, severe headache and stiff neck, the older man who suddenly finds his right field of vision going dim, the pack-a-day smoker who wakes up and realizes that the left side of his body is weak or numb—they all have markedly different symptoms, but all may be experiencing stroke. Stroke's symptoms occur throughout the body, but stroke itself occurs in the brain. Stroke is essentially a brain injury—an injury caused by the damage or death of brain cells, or neurons. Its effects are so widespread because neurons are responsible for sending the messages that control nearly every function in the body.

Neurons require lots of energy to perform their many functions. Blood rich in oxygen and other nutrients to fuel the brain is delivered twenty-four hours a day via an elaborate system of blood vessels. All told, the brain, which makes up only 2 percent of the adult body's weight, receives about 20 percent of the body's oxygen and 15 percent of the heart's output of fresh blood at rest, and, in the fasting state, consumes up to 100 percent of the liver's output of glucose, or blood sugar. The brain does not store oxygen or glucose and cannot function when it is deprived of them. As a result, if the brain's blood supply is disrupted, even for a short period of time, brain cells can become injured or die, affecting the body functions for which they were responsible.

What Happens During a Brain Attack

During a stroke, the blood supply to a part of the brain is interrupted by a blockage of a blood vessel, or a rupture of a blood vessel, sending blood into brain tissue and injuring or killing neurons in that area of the brain. The damage that results depends on the cause, severity, and location of the stroke. A person who has had a stroke on the right side of his or her brain, for example, may have difficulty moving the left side of the body or may experience visual problems or problems with perception. Someone who has had a stroke on the left side of his or her brain may have difficulty moving the right side of the body or may be unable to speak or to understand spoken or written language. In other words, injury to the brain can have repercussions throughout the body—and beyond. In addition to causing paralysis and other physical symptoms, stroke can affect language and communication abilities, perception, emotions, thinking, reasoning, and memory. It can even alter personality.

Stroke's consequences range from no discernible long-term effects to death—and everything in between. Some initial deficits resolve on their own or with rehabilitation. Other deficits may remain. Although we tend to think of stroke as a great physical debilitator—perhaps the most familiar deficit is paralysis or weakness of the leg, face, or arm, generally on one side of the body—I've found that the speech, cognitive, and emotional symptoms of stroke can be among the most trying for some stroke survivors and their families. Imagine the frustration of being unable to tell someone you need a glass of water, or not remembering the steps involved in getting dressed, or laughing or crying uncontrollably in public. The frustration and embarrassment may intensify if you or your loved ones don't understand that these deficits and behaviors are direct consequences of stroke.

Stroke's effects are so wide ranging because stroke is an injury to the brain, the master electronic control center of the entire body. These effects vary depending on the location and severity of this brain injury. Different areas of the brain are associated with control of different functions. The brain is divided into two hemispheres, or halves, which are associated with the control of movement and sensation on the opposite side of the body. Each hemisphere is also responsible for other functions and skills. The most highly developed, or dominant, hemisphere, for example, is associated with speech and language. In most people, this is the left side of the brain. Stroke can occur in either or both hemispheres, as well as in other areas of the brain.

Physical Effects

The physical effects of stroke are often the most obvious. One of the most common is weakness, paralysis, or lack of coordination of the leg, face, or arm on one side of the body. (Weakness on one side of the body is known as *hemiparesis;* paralysis on one side as *hemiplegia.*) Other physical effects include a lack of feeling and position on one side of the body (a condition known as *hemianesthesia*), difficulty swallowing, and visual problems, including defective vision or blindness in half of one or both eyes (*hemianopia*).

Cognitive Effects

Although the physical effects are the most obvious, the cognitive effects can be the most disturbing. These depend on whether the injury occurred in the dominant or nondominant hemisphere of the brain. Injuries to the brain's dominant hemisphere can result in difficulty understanding or using spoken or written language. This is known as *aphasia,* and it comes in many forms. Some people, for instance, have difficulty only with written speech; others have difficulty understanding syntax, or repeating words or sentences. Other potential problems include an inability to name objects (*anomia*), an inability to write properly (*agraphia*), confusion between left and right, an inability to identify specific fingers, and the inability to use an object or perform a task without loss of perception about the object's use or the goal of the task (*ideomotor apraxia*).

If the nondominant hemisphere is injured, the cognitive effects could include an inability to copy geometric shapes and patterns (*constructional apraxia*), impairment of spatial organization, difficulty dressing, and an inability to recognize music.

Damage to both hemispheres can affect short- and long-term memory. It can, for example, affect immediate recall (your ability to recall or repeat information after a few seconds), short-term memory (your memory of day-to-day events such as what you had for breakfast this morning), recent memory (your ability to learn new material and recall it after minutes, hours, or days), or remote memory (recollections such as historical facts and teachers' names). In some instances, it will affect only one type of memory; in others, several.

Emotional and Behavioral Effects

Stroke can also result in emotional and behavioral changes, including personality changes. It can reduce inhibitions, make someone act impulsively, decrease motivation, affect self-control and patience, and cause irritability.

It can also affect a person's control of his or her emotions, causing him or her to laugh or cry spontaneously, sometimes at inappropriate times. Not surprisingly, stroke can also trigger depression.

THE PREVENTIVE POWER OF KNOWLEDGE

Stroke is often unforeseen and poorly understood—which is why our greatest weapon against stroke is knowledge. I hope the information in this chapter—and in this book—will demystify stroke and give you power not just over fear, but over stroke itself. As you learn about the mechanics of stroke and its underlying causes, you will see that it often is not the sudden occurrence it appears to be. You'll see that there are steps you can take to keep your life stroke-free.

Teaching patients is one of the most enjoyable roles of a physician. There are several reasons why I do my best to take whatever time is required to make my patients fully informed about their condition.

First, I consider myself my patients' advocate, which means I feel a responsibility to give them whatever support is going to help them cope with their problems, whether medical or emotional. One of my most important advocacy functions is giving patients the peace of mind that comes with having their medical condition fully and clearly explained.

Second, it's therapeutic for patients to have the tools to overcome their fear of stroke. One of the greatest casualties of some of today's managed care medicine, with its emphasis on bottom-line cost-benefit analysis, is the patient's peace of mind, which is seldom factored into outcome studies. The result is that doctors are encouraged to treat bodies, not the whole person. Both the patient and the doctor lose when this happens. The less anxiety patients experience about their condition, the faster they can recuperate and heal—which is what every doctor wants.

When Mary, a thirty-eight-year-old attorney, came to see me, she was complaining of severe headaches and dizzy spells that can sometimes be a symptom of an impending stroke or other serious brain lesion. I examined her and took a detailed history. I discovered that although Mary had never had migraines, she was up for partnership in her firm that year and was worried about the outcome of a case she'd been working on for months. It also became apparent that her headaches usually occurred at the same time of day.

Mary was one of those people who had usually thrived on stress and couldn't believe that it might be contributing to her headaches. She became convinced that she had a brain tumor or an aneurysm. The more she worried about this possibility, the worse her headaches became. It had gotten to the point where she couldn't function at work. She was so anxious that she was also having trouble sleeping through the night.

Based on her history and symptoms, it wasn't likely that Mary had a brain tumor, aneurysm, or other serious brain abnormality. To be on the safe side, we did some imaging studies of her head. When the tests came back clean, Mary was hugely relieved. I spent an hour or so reviewing the studies with her and explaining why I believed her headaches were primarily tension-related, rather than from a more serious underlying condition. I suggested some simple stress-reduction techniques, including some she could do in her office each afternoon. When she came back to see me a week later, she reported that the frequency and intensity of her headaches had fallen off dramatically, and she was sleeping better, too. A month later, her headaches had subsided altogether.

Someone at an HMO reviewing this case might argue that the imaging study made no difference to the patient's outcome, so that there was no cost benefit to the study, or even to doing a detailed history and exam. Of course, what that kind of bottom-line analysis overlooks is that in this case Mary's peace of mind was critical to her ability to get better and get back into her life.

Finally, I believe in educating patients because an informed patient is a better diagnostic and treatment partner for me. Despite all the advances we've made in stroke medicine in the past decades, so much of what we still do is wade through the unknown. Although I have a lot of technology at my disposal, my best source of information about any individual case is my patient. The better educated a patient is about stroke, the more I can learn from him or her in terms of personal history, signs, and symptoms.

My judgments, like those of any doctor, are based on a mix of hard data, past experience, and intuition. What I've learned is that better-educated patients have more evolved intuition about their own bodies—which makes them more valuable allies in puzzling out their problems and deciding on treatment. Whenever I'm facing a difficult decision with a patient about what course of action to take, I listen to the patient's instincts about what his or her body needs. Being able to listen to and hear my patients is one of my most important faculties as a doctor. And giving them the information they need to express and articulate their symptoms, feelings, and even their hunches is one of my most crucial tasks.

THE ANATOMY OF STROKE

Few people really think about the possible ramifications of stroke, much less its mechanics and causes. Even the medical profession has been slow to understand stroke. Although we have known for years that stroke is the result of blockage or bleeding involving the brain, only in the past fifty years have we gained an understanding of the functional changes that accompany those two types of injuries and of their underlying causes. Only in the past twenty-five years, since the development of computed tomography, or CT, scans, have we been able to diagnose the type of stroke with great precision. Only in the past fifteen years have we begun to identify the various risk factors for each type of stroke. Our knowledge of stroke is still evolving. New scanning techniques are allowing us to see for the first time the biochemical changes that occur in the brain. New risk factors are being identified. With this information, new treatments and preventive measures are being developed, and the death rate from stroke has declined significantly.

Here's what we now know happens inside the brain during a brain attack and the major factors that cause or contribute to stroke. There are two major types of stroke: ischemic stroke and hemorrhagic stroke. Ischemic stroke is caused by a reduction in the flow of blood to the brain. Hemorrhagic stroke results from bleeding in or around the brain.

ISCHEMIC STROKE

Ischemic stroke accounts for about 80 percent of all strokes. Think of it as a siege of the brain. The brain needs oxygenated blood to function. This blood is supplied by a vast network of arteries, a series of roads. When passage through these vessels is cut off, say by a clot, the brain starves in much the same way a city starves when an enemy cuts off its access to the roads that connect it to the outside world. Deprived of oxygen, brain cells eventually die. The body, like the city, is left disabled or destroyed.

This assault on the brain, like a wartime siege, generally is the res
longtime buildup of enemy activity—in most cases, involving the bioo᠆
vessels or heart. Among the contributing factors are atherosclerosis (often
referred to as hardening of the arteries), hypertension (high blood pressure),
and various heart conditions. Atherosclerosis contributes to stroke by narrowing blood vessels, reducing blood flow, and contributing to the formation of blood clots. Hypertension causes arteries to thicken and constrict.
Certain heart conditions can generate clots or affect the body's overall blood
supply.

The lack of blood supply is the crucial factor in ischemic stroke. To
understand how blood flow to the brain can be interrupted, you need to
understand how it is supplied. The brain receives its blood from the carotid
and vertebral arteries. The common carotid arteries run up from either side
of the front of the neck. Near the head, they branch into the external
carotid arteries and the internal carotid arteries, which ultimately supply
blood to the front and upper regions of the brain. The smaller vertebral
arteries run up the back of the neck and supply blood to the back and bottom portions of the brain. Within the skull, the carotid and vertebral arteries branch off and break into smaller and smaller arteries and capillaries that
bring blood to all parts of the brain.

When the flow of blood through any of these arteries or capillaries is
obstructed, an area of brain tissue becomes *ischemic,* or deprived of oxygen
and nutrients. If blood is not restored promptly, the tissue dies. This dead
tissue is known as an *infarct.* In fact, another medical term for ischemic
stroke is *cerebral infarction.* Cerebral infarction, or brain attack, like
myocardial infarction, or heart attack, requires prompt medical attention.

Most ischemic strokes are caused by a blood clot, or *thrombus,* that
blocks a vessel that supplies blood to an area of the brain (you may hear this
referred to as *thrombotic stroke*) or by an *embolus,* a clot originating elsewhere in the body that travels to and becomes lodged in a vessel that supplies blood to the brain (this may be referred to as *embolic stroke*). Ischemic
stroke can also result when circulatory problems or a buildup of atherosclerotic plaque reduce the overall blood flow to the brain (this is sometimes
called *hypoperfusion*).

If the blood supply is interrupted only briefly and symptoms disappear
within twenty-four hours, the episode is known as a *transient ischemic*

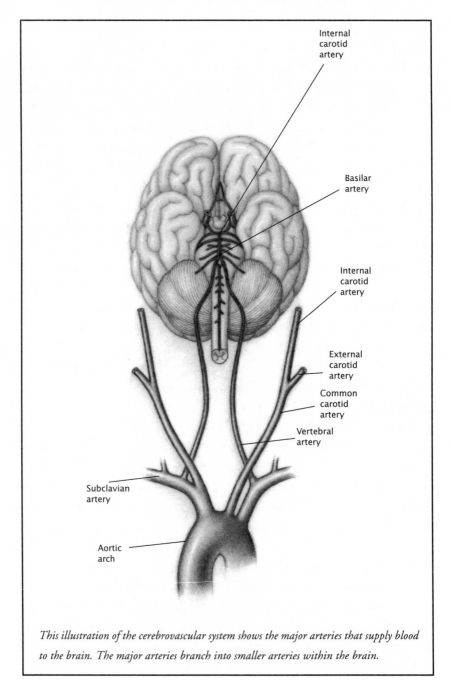

Internal
carotid
artery

Basilar
artery

Internal
carotid
artery

External
carotid
artery

Common
carotid
artery

Vertebral
artery

Subclavian
artery

Aortic
arch

This illustration of the cerebrovascular system shows the major arteries that supply blood to the brain. The major arteries branch into smaller arteries within the brain.

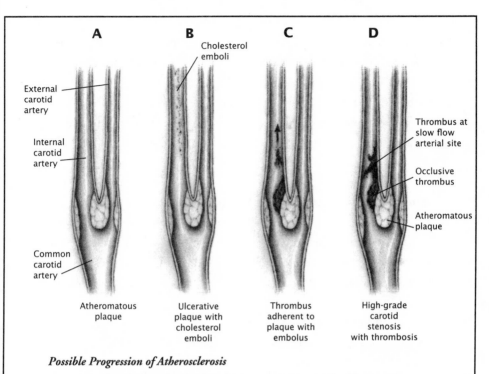

A   **B**   **C**   **D**

Cholesterol
emboli

External
carotid
artery

Internal
carotid
artery

Thrombus at
slow flow
arterial site

Occlusive
thrombus

Atheromatous
plaque

Common
carotid
artery

Atheromatous
plaque

Ulcerative
plaque with
cholesterol
emboli

Thrombus
adherent to
plaque with
embolus

High-grade
carotid
stenosis
with thrombosis

Possible Progression of Atherosclerosis

A. *Atherosclerotic plaque (in white) has built up on the inner walls of the carotid artery.*

B. *The plaque buildup has begun to release small, mobile pieces of cholesterol into the bloodstream.*

C. *A blood clot adheres to the plaque buildup on the artery walls and a piece of clot breaks loose.*

D. *Plaque buildup and a clot significantly narrow the carotid artery, a situation known as high-grade stenosis. In some instances, the narrowing completely blocks the artery (occlusion).*

attack, or *TIA.* These events, sometimes called "mini-strokes," are a major risk factor for ischemic stroke and should not be ignored. TIAs precede between 20 and 40 percent of ischemic strokes and offer a clear sign that something is wrong. The temporary numbness that Jack experienced was likely a TIA. If he had sought medical attention instead of ignoring the symptoms, he might have been able to prevent the ischemic stroke he suffered two days later.

Jack had several risk factors for ischemic stroke: high blood pressure, smoking, and a poor diet. It's highly likely he also had atherosclerosis. Any of these factors could have caused his stroke. An examination could probably pinpoint the exact cause. This would enable us to identify the type of stroke he had.

Stroke specialists generally classify ischemic stroke by cause or mechanism. These strokes generally originate in the large blood vessels supplying the brain, the small blood vessels of the brain, the heart, or in the blood itself.

Atherosclerotic ischemic strokes, those caused by atherosclerosis (hardening of the arteries), are responsible for about 25 percent of all strokes. Atherosclerosis can appear anywhere in the body. It is likely to cause stroke when it affects the arteries that deliver blood to the brain, including such large arteries as the carotid and vertebral arteries, and smaller cerebral arteries and arterioles.

Cardioembolic ischemic strokes, those caused by emboli that originate in the heart and travel to the blood vessels in the brain, account for about 25 percent of all strokes. These clots can result from a number of conditions, ranging from valvular heart problems and diseases to rhythm disorders to heart attack, heart failure, and diseases of the heart muscle itself.

Hypertension, or high blood pressure, which affects the small blood vessels, is linked to several types of brain lesions, including **lacunar infarctions,** small areas of dead tissue deep in the brain in areas supplied by small blood vessels. Lacunar infarctions cause about 20 percent of all strokes.

Other ischemic strokes can be caused by a variety of conditions, including disorders that affect the blood vessels like arteritis (inflammation of the blood vessels) and abnormalities of the blood that thicken it or make it more likely to clot. The most well-known blood abnormality is sickle-cell disease, an inherited disorder in which red blood cells develop a curved, sickle shape. Diseases that affect the actual composition of the blood, the number of red blood cells or platelets, for example, can also cause ischemic stroke. Approximately 10 percent of all strokes fall into this catchall category. A complete list of the conditions that can cause ischemic stroke is included on pages 26–28.

Stroke Subtypes by Percentage

ISCHEMIC*

Atherosclerotic	25 percent
Cardioembolic	25 percent
Lacunar infarction	20 percent
Other (blood disorders, etc.)	10 percent

HEMORRHAGIC

Subarachnoid hemorrhage	5–10 percent
Intracerebral hemorrhage	10–15 percent

*In some cases, the cause of ischemic stroke cannot be determined. Because of this uncertainty, the percentages included here are based on known statistics, the uncertainty factor, and my own best judgment.

HEMORRHAGIC STROKE

Although lack of oxygen and nutrients plays some role in hemorrhagic stroke, the condition is more of a flood than a siege. Hemorrhagic stroke is caused by the rupture or leakage of a blood vessel in the brain, which does, of course, interrupt blood supply to the portion of the brain supplied by that vessel. The outpouring of blood also floods the area of the brain where the leak occurred, displacing and putting pressure on brain tissue and affecting its function. The flood also may cause surrounding arteries to spasm, ultimately resulting in ischemic stroke.

Many floods result from the leaking or breaking of a dam, which is often caused by some weakness within the dam. Similarly, most hemorrhagic strokes are caused by the rupture of a blood vessel within the brain, generally one that has been weakened by an aneurysm, malformation, or the continuous effects of hypertension. And as you might expect, brain hemorrhage can also be caused by a sudden injury or blow to the head.

Unlike ischemic strokes, which stroke specialists classify by mechanism or cause, brain hemorrhages are classified based on the location of the hemorrhage, which relates to mechanism. There are five types of brain hemorrhage: epidural hematoma, subdural hematoma, subarachnoid hemorrhage, intracerebral hemorrhage, and intraventricular hemorrhage. Because the first two, which occur in the outermost part of the brain, are generally the result of head injuries and the fifth, intraventricular hemorrhage, occurs deep in the brain as the result of other brain hemorrhages, they are not considered stroke subtypes and are not included in stroke statistics.

Epidural hematoma is a collection of blood between the skull and the outermost membrane of the brain, the *dura*.

Subdural hematoma is a collection of blood between the dura and the underlying brain. Both are largely the result of head injuries that result in the rupture of an artery or vein.

Intraventricular hemorrhage occurs within the small cavities deep within the brain. It is usually an extension of intracerebral or subarachnoid hemorrhage, the two subtypes of hemorrhagic stroke.

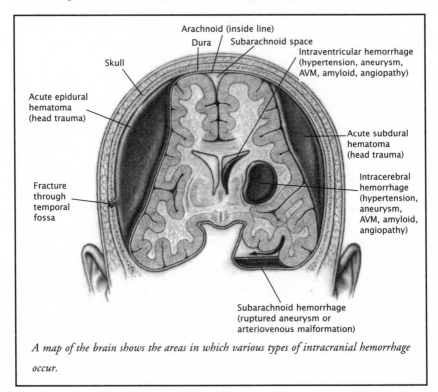

A map of the brain shows the areas in which various types of intracranial hemorrhage occur.

Subarachnoid Hemorrhage

Subarachnoid hemorrhage, which causes 5 to 10 percent of all strokes, occurs under or within the arachnoid space, between the surface of the brain and the skull. Women are more likely than men to experience subarachnoid hemorrhage, which often manifests itself as a sudden, severe headache unlike any previously felt. Several conditions can cause bleeding in this area, including the rupture of an aneurysm (the ballooning of a weakened area of a blood vessel wall) or a blood vessel malformation; head injury, hypertension, and blood disorders. The most common cause is the rupture of an intracranial aneurysm.

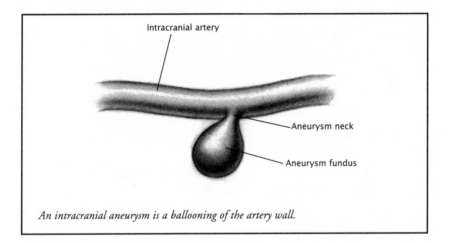

Intracranial artery

Aneurysm neck

Aneurysm fundus

An intracranial aneurysm is a ballooning of the artery wall.

Intracerebral Hemorrhage

Intracerebral hemorrhage occurs within the brain and, like subarachnoid hemorrhage, is often signaled by a severe headache. It accounts for 10 to 15 percent of all strokes and is most often caused by chronic hypertension. In fact, hypertension is responsible for about 60 percent of all intracerebral hemorrhages. Other causes include ruptured intracranial aneurysms, vascular malformations, complications of anticoagulant (blood-thinning) therapy, blood disorders, and head injury.

I discuss the specific causes of stroke in more detail in chapter 3. They include the following:

Underlying Causes of Stroke

ISCHEMIC STROKE

Atherosclerotic Ischemic Stroke

Atherosclerosis

Cardioembolic Ischemic Stroke

Atrial fibrillation

Sick sinus syndrome

Other major rhythm disturbances

Mitral valve prolapse (severe)

Mitral annulus calcification

Calcific aortic stenosis

Mechanical or replacement heart valve

Congestive heart failure

Recent heart attack (myocardial infarction)

Endocarditis (infective or nonbacterial thrombotic)

Clot in heart (intracardiac thrombus)

Ventricular aneurysm

Rheumatic heart disease

Congenital heart diseases

Cardiomyopathy

Patent foramen ovale

Hypokinetic/akinetic heart segment

Cardiac procedures, including surgery, catheterization, and
    arteriography

Atrial myxoma

Cardiac fibroelastoma

Pulmonary vein thrombosis

Pulmonary arteriovenous malformation

Lacunar Infarction

Hypertension

Other Ischemic Stroke

Sickle-cell disease

Infectious arteritis (caused by bacterial, fungal, tuberculous
meningitides or diseases such as tertiary syphilis, malaria,
Lyme disease, rickettsial diseases, mucormycosis, aspergillosis,
trichinosis, schistosomiasis, herpes zoster, basal meningitis)

Noninfectious arteritis (caused by systemic lupus erythematosus,
polyarteritis nodosa, granulomatous angiitis, temporal arteritis,
Takayasu's arteritis, Behçet's disease, Wegener's granulomatosis,
Sjögren's syndrome, sarcoidosis, irradiation arteritis, drug use
and abuse including cocaine, heroin, amphetamine,
phencyclidine, and LSD)

Polycythemia

Thrombocythemia

Thrombocytopenic purpura

Dysproteinemia

Antiphospholipid antibody syndromes

Leukemia

Disseminated intravascular coagulation

Sneddon's syndrome

Protein C and protein S deficiency

Antithrombin III deficiency

Resistance to activated protein C

Vasospasm (migraine)

Fibromuscular dysplasia

Carotid artery dissection

Brain or neck radiation

Homocystinuria

Moyamoya disease

Fabry's disease

Pseudoxanthoma elasticum

HEMORRHAGIC STROKE

Subarachnoid Hemorrhage

Intracranial aneurysm

Arteriovenous malformation

Anticoagulant therapy/Thrombolytic therapy

Disseminated intravascular coagulation (often associated with
leukemia or thrombocytopenia)

Head trauma

Cortical vein and dural sinus thrombosis

Bleeding disorders (for example, hemophilia)

Arterial dissection

Brain tumor

Cerebral vasculitis

Spinal lesions

Drugs, including alcohol abuse and cocaine abuse

Intracerebral Hemorrhage

Hypertension

Arteriovenous malformation

Intracranial aneurysm

Anticoagulant therapy/Thrombolytic therapy

Antiplatelet agents

Bleeding disorders (for example, hemophilia)

Cerebral arteritis

Thrombocytopenia

Cerebral amyloid angiopathy

Head trauma

Brain tumors

Arterial dissection

Moyamoya disease

Venous thrombosis

Infection

Abscess

Drugs, including cocaine, phenylpropanolamine, alcohol,
and heroin

A FINAL WORD

Although ischemic stroke and hemorrhagic stroke are both medical emergencies, they are, in some ways, almost total opposites. One is caused by not

enough blood, the other by too much—or, more precisely, too much in the wrong place. With few exceptions, including hypertension, arteritis, and endocarditis, they have different underlying conditions. They are often signaled by different symptoms. And they require very different treatments while they are in progress. The blood-thinning drugs that could save the life of a person with ischemic stroke could actually worsen the condition of a person with hemorrhagic stroke, perhaps at the cost of his or her life. To put it bluntly, you don't fix a clogged pipe the same way you fix a leaky one.

The development and use of the CT scan and other imaging techniques have greatly improved our ability to differentiate between the two types of stroke and, consequently, to provide appropriate treatment. You should be aware that some doctors do not verbally distinguish between the two types. Although the term *stroke* can refer to either type, some doctors use it only when describing ischemic stroke. Many doctors still refer to both types of stroke as *cerebrovascular accident,* a blanket clinical term.

In a similar manner, although some stroke specialists use the term *cerebral hemorrhage* to refer to intracerebral hemorrhage, some practitioners and many in the media use the term to refer to any hemorrhage, or bleeding, in the head, including that caused by trauma as well as by either type of hemorrhagic stroke.

You now know the differences among these stroke types and subtypes and are ready to assess your risk for each.

3

Assessing Your Risk of Stroke

Nobody likes to take tests, but I can tell you that taking the self-assessment quiz in this chapter can add years—even decades—to your productive life. In less than an hour, you'll have a comprehensive picture of your risk level for stroke, and most important, you will have taken the first step toward preventing your stroke from ever occurring.

This risk assessment tool has not been available until now. It's based on decades of research, both here at Mayo Clinic and around the world at other leading stroke centers. Our goal has been to distill a wealth of research data and high-tech computation from epidemiological studies into a simple quiz that anyone could complete with a sheet of paper and a pencil in under an hour.

HOW THIS SELF-ASSESSMENT TEST EVOLVED

The setting for this story is Mayo Clinic in Rochester, Minnesota. At first glance, this large, world-class medical center seems out of place in a small rural community. In fact, the Rochester community is a hybrid of the approximately 80,000 permanent residents and a parallel population of visitors who are either patients at Mayo or family members of patients. This makes for a remarkably eclectic community of people from around the world. In a typical day a physician might treat a farmer, an electrician, or a schoolteacher from the surrounding area, as well as a visiting dignitary from the Middle East, a Broadway actor, or a Russian poet. What's most compelling about these individuals, from a medical point of view, is how disease remains the great equalizer. Although their ethnic and economic backgrounds may affect their specific risk factors, all of them face the threat of stroke, and all of them need to consider certain lifestyle adjustments—or face the same surgical or drug interventions—in order to stay healthy.

The relatively small community of Rochester residents has played a disproportionately large and dramatic role in the history of epidemiological medicine. Mayo Clinic's Rochester Epidemiology Project has charted the health of the entire population of Olmsted County, Minnesota, for more than forty years. This one-of-a-kind database provides us with rare insight into long-term trends in disease incidence and specific information about how different variables affect disease risk in combination and over time. This ongoing study, which was made possible by the foresight of many others at Mayo Clinic who came before me, is now considered a gold standard of population-based epidemiological studies.

The study has been a wellspring of revelations about what causes stroke. My colleagues and I have tapped this resource for numerous studies and research papers, but each paper presents only a piece of the puzzle. One study focuses on the role of atherosclerosis as a risk factor, while another focuses on the role of hypertension, and so on. We wanted to assemble all the pieces of this puzzle and come up with a comprehensive and simple way to assess risk.

When I began serving as head of the Mayo Stroke Center six years ago, my colleagues and I took a hard look at the information the center had accumulated in its four decades of research. We were struck by how the cumulative data we had at our fingertips could enable us to assess stroke risk accurately and to take calculated steps to prevent stroke—insight that could shift the approach to stroke from reactive to preventive.

Devising an accurate risk assessment tool was problematic, because of the complexity of the many variables and interactions that go into calculating stroke risk. We initially decided to put the assessment in the form of a computer program to assess risk for ischemic stroke, the most common type. We boiled down much of Mayo research into a short list of questions that could be answered by doctors or patients and then fed a massive amount of data into the computer. The program used the data to calculate that person's percentage risk of having an ischemic stroke in any time frame—one, five, or ten years, for example.

Even as we put the finishing touches on the program, it became apparent: The computer program would help health care providers, insurers, and the government make important decisions about the value and cost-effectiveness of treating major risk factors in the community. But it wasn't a practical tool for the millions of individuals who are at risk of stroke and who need to adopt a prevention program immediately. The computer program had other limitations as well. It failed to take into account the subtypes of ischemic stroke and, by design, did not address risk factors for hemorrhagic stroke. It offered no guidance on how to address the risk factors it identified. Just as in other aspects of medicine, we had developed a high-tech tool that was only a partial solution to the problem.

That realization was the driving force behind this book and the assessment included here. We wanted to provide patients with all the information they need to know about stroke risk—to create an assessment that measures overall stroke risk and the risk for each stroke subtype and to outline the steps patients can take to address each of their personal risk factors. We went back to the drawing board and developed a sixty-question test that does just that. The test is easy to complete and paints a clear, individualized picture of stroke risk. What's more, it directs you to the part of the book that tells you what you can do about it.

We're excited about this new approach to risk assessment. It's simple and comprehensive, and it provides you with information you can find nowhere else. Along with Mayo Clinic research included in the computer assessment, the assessment in this book takes into account data from studies from other populations and medical centers and those we have collaborated on or conducted around the world, tempered by my judgment and that of my colleagues.

In addition to the standard questions about age, gender, and heart health you may have seen in other stroke assessments, you'll find questions about your eating habits, exercise habits, and mental health—factors that increasingly appear to play a role in stroke risk and factors over which you have some control. The assessment will also enable you to determine, for the first time, the subtype or subtypes of stroke for which you are at greatest risk.

This is critical information to have when it comes to devising a prevention plan. Since the system we've created to assess the various risk factors takes into account not only the relative risk each factor confers for each stroke subtype but also the frequency at which each subtype occurs, you will get an accurate picture of your overall stroke risk.

I explain the various risk factors and the research behind them later in this chapter. You're welcome to read about all of them. Since each person's risk profile is individual, and not all risk factors apply to all people, I present the assessment first. That way you can determine which risk factors apply to you and read only about those factors if you so choose.

A WORD ABOUT RISK FACTORS

The risk factors for stroke are numerous and varied, often directly related to the causes of stroke. Some of these risks, like calendar age and gender, cannot be altered or controlled. Others, like smoking and eating a high-fat, high-cholesterol diet, can be reduced or eliminated. Risk factors do not actually dictate whether a person will have a stroke. They indicate an increased likelihood of having a stroke and the subtype or subtypes of stroke a person is most likely to experience. A person with few risk factors can have a stroke, while a person with many risk factors can escape that fate. Statistically, the person with many risk factors, particularly in certain combinations, is more likely to have a stroke than the person with few risk factors.

The number and combination of risk factors you have is not etched in stone. If, when you complete the assessment, you find that you are at high risk of having a stroke, don't panic. Even bad news can be good news. The risk assessment is not a deterministic prophesy of things to come. It is simply a snapshot of your risk at a particular time. Although you cannot change such risk factors as age, gender, and family history, you can reduce or eliminate others by taking the preventive steps outlined in chapters 4 and 5. If you take action to address modifiable risk factors, you may find that your overall stroke risk has decreased the next time you complete the assessment.

Finally, you need to realize that changes in stroke risk go both ways. Just as the actions you take and the choices you make can reduce your risk, they can also increase it. Your risk can also increase for reasons outside your control. For example, you will get older. In addition, we cannot currently stop the inevitable development of certain genetically influenced conditions that increase risk. This doesn't mean you have no control over your stroke risk. You simply need to do everything you can do to modify—or prevent—the risk factors over which you have control. Even if you are at low risk for stroke, you can and should take action—in this case to keep your risk low and, perhaps, cheat Father Time a little. The information in chapter 5, "The Stroke-Free for Life Prevention Plan," will help you accomplish this goal.

HOW THE ASSESSMENT IS STRUCTURED

The assessment begins with a pretest—a series of eight yes-or-no questions. If you answer yes to any of these questions, you should see your doctor or a stroke specialist in short order, because you may be in imminent danger of having a stroke. Don't spend time completing the assessment questionnaire.

The questionnaire itself consists of sixty numbered, yes-or-no questions, organized into seven categories: personal information, lifestyle information, medications, neurological information, cardiac information, other medical information, and family history. Each question is followed by the heading and page number or page numbers on which the risk factor or factors are discussed later in the chapter and seven columns containing numerical scores. The numbers in the seven columns indicate the degree of risk the factor conveys for the six stroke subtypes (atherosclerotic, cardioembolic, lacunar, other ischemic, subarachnoid hemorrhage, and intracerebral hemorrhage) and for overall stroke risk.

HOW TO COMPLETE THE ASSESSMENT

To complete the assessment, you'll need a pen or pencil and a lined sheet of paper. You may also want a calculator. On the top of the left side of your paper, write "Risk Factors." On the top of the right side of your paper, write the headings of the six stroke subtypes that appear on the questionnaire in the book that correspond to columns A, B, C, D, E, F. You may also wish to make a heading for the overall risk index, or total score, although you don't need to do this. (There's an easier way to find your overall risk index score.) You may want to draw vertical columns for each heading. When you complete this, you are ready to take the assessment.

Question	A	B	C	D	E	F	Total
Q1	2	2	1	1	0	1	
Q4	2	1	1	0	0	0	
Q8	4	3	3	2	2	3	
Q15	2	0	0	0	0	0	
Q17	3	1	1	0	0	0	
Q44	5	3	6	3	0	5	
Q46	5	0	2	0	0	0	
Q57	0	0	1	0	0	1	
Totals	23	10	15	6	2	10	66

This is an example of what your worksheet should look like.

Read the questions in order, and do not skip any. For each question to which your answer is yes, write the question number (Q1, Q2, etc.) and name of the risk factor on the left side of your paper, then copy the six (or seven) corresponding numerical scores in the columns you created on the right side of the paper, making sure that each number goes under the correct heading.

If you have one of the conditions listed, such as hypertension, diabetes mellitus, or a high cholesterol level, but that condition is under control as a result of lifestyle and/or medical treatment, you should answer the corresponding question yes. Later in the chapter, I'll tell you how to adjust your score to account for your treatment.

Completing the assessment should take anywhere from ten minutes to an hour, depending on the number of questions that apply to you and your knowledge of your medical history. If you do not have information about your medical history, complete the questions you can answer, for instance, those in the first three sections. To answer some of the questions dealing with certain medical conditions, you may find it helpful to refer to the risk factor discussion later in the chapter, where each condition is defined and explained (see page number and heading column). You may need to get a copy of your medical record or consult with your doctor to complete some of the questions. You may also need to check with one or more family members to answer the questions about your family history.

THE ASSESSMENT

Before you complete the assessment, answer the eight questions that follow. I call them the "Scary Eight" because they indicate urgent stroke risk. These are the first questions I ask my patients when I begin to determine their stroke risk. If you don't understand the medical terminology used in the question, turn to the page number(s) provided for an explanation of the condition(s). The term "recently" in questions two through eight refers to a time period within the past few months.

The Scary Eight

If you answer yes to any of these questions, see your doctor or stroke specialist immediately. You may be in imminent danger of having a stroke.

1. Have you had one or more TIAs/minor ischemic strokes within the past four weeks? (See page 81.)
2. Have you recently had a TIA/minor ischemic stroke and been diagnosed with atrial fibrillation? (See page 55.)
3. Have you recently had a TIA/minor ischemic stroke and recently been diagnosed with congestive heart failure? (See page 60.)
4. Have you recently had a TIA/minor ischemic stroke and have you been diagnosed with any of the following heart conditions: sick sinus syndrome (see page 79), mitral or aortic heart valve disease (see page 72), endocarditis (see page 65), ventricular aneurysm (see page 84), clot in the heart (see page 59), prosthetic heart valve (see page 77)?
5. Have you recently had a TIA/minor ischemic stroke and been diagnosed with high-grade carotid stenosis (narrowing)? (See page 54.)
6. Have you recently had a TIA/minor ischemic stroke and been diagnosed with very high blood pressure (greater than 200/110 mm Hg)? (See page 67.)

7. Have you recently experienced a warning leak from an intracranial aneurysm (see page 69) or vascular malformation in the brain (see page 83)?
8. Have you recently experienced symptoms of an intracranial aneurysm (or, less urgently, a vascular malformation) other than a warning leak or rupture? (See pages 69 and 83.)

Your Personal Risk Assessment Quiz

Read each question below and record the scores of any yes answers on your paper as described in "How to Complete the Assessment."

| Question | Heading (Page #) | ISCHEMIC | | | | HEMORRHAGIC | | Overall Risk Index |
		A (Athero)	B (Cardiac)	C (Lacunar)	D (Other)	E (SAH)	F (ICH)	
PERSONAL INFORMATION								
Q1. Are you male?	Gender (67)	2	2	1	1	0	1	7
Q2. Are you female?	Gender (67)	0	0	0	0	3	0	3
Q3. Are you African American?	Race (77)	1	0	2	1	0	2	6
Q4. Are you Caucasian?	Race (77)	2	1	1	0	0	0	4
Q5. Are you of Asian descent?	Race (77)	0	0	0	0	2	2	4
Q6. Are you 45–54?	Age (51)	1	1	1	0	0	1	4
Q7. Are you 55–64?	Age (51)	2	2	2	1	1	2	10
Q8. Are you 65–74?	Age (51)	4	3	3	2	2	3	17
Q9. Are you 75 or older?	Age (51)	8	5	5	3	3	6	30
Q10. Do you have a body mass index greater than or equal to 25? (See Appendix A)	Body Mass Index (56)	2	2	2	1	0	0	7
Q11. Do you have a body mass index less than or equal to 19? (See Appendix A)	Body Mass Index (56)	0	0	0	0	2	0	2
LIFESTYLE INFORMATION								
Q12. Do you smoke or have you smoked within the last five years?	Smoking (80)	5	2	2	1	5	2	17

| Question | Heading (Page #) | ISCHEMIC | | | | HEMORRHAGIC | | Overall |
		A (Athero)	B (Cardiac)	C (Lacunar)	D (Other)	E (SAH)	F (ICH)	Risk Index
LIFESTYLE INFORMATION								
Q13. If you don't smoke, have you spent a significant amount of time around a smoker in the last five years?	Smoking (80)	2	1	1	1	2	1	8
Q14. Do you drink alcohol excessively (3 or more ounces per day)?	Alcohol (51)	0	1	0	0	3	2	6
Q15. Do you abstain from alcohol?	Alcohol (51)	2	0	0	0	0	0	2
Q16. Do you eat a diet high in salt?	Diet (62)	1	0	2	0	0	2	5
Q17. Do you eat a diet high in cholesterol and saturated fat (high in meat, eggs, and dairy products)?	Diet (62)	3	1	1	0	0	0	5
Q18. Do you eat a diet that is low in fruits and vegetables?	Diet (62)	4	1	1	0	0	0	6
Q19. Are you under a great deal of chronic stress, do you suffer from an anxiety disorder, or do you regularly take medications with stimulant effects?	Stress and/or Stimulant Drugs (81)	1	0	2	0	2	2	7
Q20. Do you exercise infrequently (less than thirty minutes three times per week)?	Exercise (65)	3	2	2	1	0	1	9

Question	Heading (Page #)	ISCHEMIC				HEMORRHAGIC		Overall Risk Index
		A (Athero)	B (Cardiac)	C (Lacunar)	D (Other)	E (SAH)	F (ICH)	
MEDICATIONS								
Q21. Do you take oral contraceptives or hormone replacement therapy?*	Oral Contraceptives/ Hormone Replacement (73)	0	2	0	1	0	0	3
Q22. Do you take any anticoagulants?	Anticoagulants (52)	0	0	0	0	4	10	14
Q23. Do you take antiplatelet agents?*	Antiplatelet Agents (53)	0	0	0	0	1	1	2
NEUROLOGICAL INFORMATION								
Q24. Have you had one or more transient ischemic attacks/minor ischemic strokes within the past year, but not within the past four weeks?	Transient Ischemic Attacks/Minor Ischemic Strokes (81)	10	10	9	7	0	0	36
Q25. Have you had one or more transient ischemic attacks/minor ischemic strokes more than one year ago?	Transient Ischemic Attacks/Minor Ischemic Strokes (81)	5	5	5	3	0	0	18
Q26. Have you ever been diagnosed with an intracranial aneurysm?	Intracranial Aneurysm (69)	0	0	0	0	5	3	8
Q27. Have you ever been diagnosed with a vascular malformation in the brain?	Vascular Malformation (83)	0	0	0	0	3	5	8

| | | ISCHEMIC | | | | HEMORRHAGIC | | |
Question	Heading (Page #)	A (Athero)	B (Cardiac)	C (Lacunar)	D (Other)	E (SAH)	F (ICH)	Overall Risk Index
CARDIAC INFORMATION								
Q28. Have you been diagnosed with atrial fibrillation?	Atrial Fibrillation (55)	0	5	0	0	0	0	5
Q29. Have you been diagnosed with sick sinus syndrome?	Sick Sinus Syndrome (79)	0	4	0	0	0	0	4
Q30. Have you been diagnosed with mitral or aortic heart valve disease?	Mitral or Aortic Heart Valve Disease (72)	0	4	0	0	0	0	4
Q31. Do you have a prosthetic heart valve?	Prosthetic Heart Valve (77)	0	5	0	0	0	0	5
Q32. Do you have congestive heart failure?	Congestive Heart Failure (60)	0	5	0	0	0	0	5
Q33. Have you had a heart attack in the last month? (Recent Heart Attack)	Recent Heart Attack (78)	0	5	0	0	0	0	5
Q34. Have you been diagnosed with endocarditis?	Endocarditis (65)	0	5	0	0	1	0	6
Q35. Have you been diagnosed with a clot in the heart?	Clot in Heart (59)	0	5	0	0	0	0	5
Q36. Have you been diagnosed with a ventricular aneurysm (aneurysm in the ventricle of the heart)?	Ventricular Aneurysm (84)	0	4	0	0	0	0	4
Q37. Have you had rheumatic heart disease?	Rheumatic Heart Disease (79)	0	5	0	0	0	0	5
Q38. Do you have any congenital heart defects?	Congenital Heart Defects (59)	0	4	0	0	0	0	4
Q39. Do you have cardiomyopathy (enlarged heart)?	Cardiomyopathy (57)	0	5	0	0	0	0	5
Q40. Do you have patent foramen ovale?	Patent Foramen Ovale (76)	0	2	0	0	0	0	2

Question	Heading (Page #)	ISCHEMIC				HEMORRHAGIC		Overall Risk Index
		A (Athero)	B (Cardiac)	C (Lacunar)	D (Other)	E (SAH)	F (ICH)	
CARDIAC INFORMATION								
Q41. Have you been diagnosed with ischemic heart disease (heart attack, angina, coronary blockage) or intermittent claudication?	Ischemic Heart Disease or Intermittent Claudication (69, 70)	3	1	0	0	0	0	4
Q42. Have you been diagnosed with a hypokinetic/ akinetic heart segment?	Hypokinetic/ Akinetic Heart Segment (68)	0	3	0	0	0	0	3
OTHER MEDICAL/NEUROLOGICAL INFORMATION								
Q43. Have you been diagnosed with a blockage or narrowing in one of the arteries in your neck?	Artery Blockage or Narrowing (54)	4	1	0	0	0	0	5
Q44. Do you have mild to moderate hypertension (between 140/90 and 179/104 mm Hg) that is unassociated with an enlarged left heart ventricle?	Hypertension (67)	5	3	6	3	0	5	22
Q45. Do you have moderate or severe hypertension (180/105 mm Hg or higher) or hypertension associated with an enlarged left heart ventricle?	Hypertension (67)	6	4	8	3	0	10	31
Q46. Do you have diabetes mellitus?	Diabetes Mellitus (61)	5	0	2	0	0	0	7
Q47. Have you been diagnosed with sickle-cell disease?	Sickle-Cell Disease (80)	0	0	0	5	0	0	5

Question	Heading (Page #)	ISCHEMIC				HEMORRHAGIC		Overall Risk Index
		A (Athero)	B (Cardiac)	C (Lacunar)	D (Other)	E (SAH)	F (ICH)	
OTHER MEDICAL NEUROLOGICAL INFORMATION								
Q48. Have you been diagnosed with arteritis?	Arteritis (54)	0	0	0	5	1	1	7
Q49. Have you been diagnosed with any of the following blood disorders: polycythemia, thrombocythemia, thrombocytopenic purpura, dysproteinemia, antiphospholipid antibody syndrome, leukemia, disseminated intravascular coagulation, or any other condition that causes your blood to clot too readily?	Disorders That Cause Increased Clotting (64)	0	0	0	5	0	0	5
Q50. Do you have hemophilia or any other condition that affects your blood's ability to clot?	Bleeding Disorders (56)	0	0	0	0	3	7	10
Q51. Have you been diagnosed with any of the following: polycystic kidney disease, coarctation of the aorta, Marfan's syndrome, Ehlers-Danlos syndrome, fibromuscular dysplasia, pseudoxanthoma elasticum, moyamoya disease, neurofibromatosis, or a pituitary tumor?	Diseases Linked to Intracranial Aneurysms (63)	0	0	0	0	3	2	5

Question	Heading (Page #)	ISCHEMIC				HEMORRHAGIC		Overall Risk Index
		A (Athero)	B (Cardiac)	C (Lacunar)	D (Other)	E (SAH)	F (ICH)	
OTHER MEDICAL/NEUROLOGICAL INFORMATION								
Q52. Do you have any of the following: a total cholesterol level above 200 mg/dL, a low-density lipoprotein level above 130 mg/dL, a triglyceride level above 200 mg/dL, or a high-density lipoprotein level below 45 mg/dL?	Cholesterol and Triglyceride Levels (58)	5	1	1	0	0	0	7
Q53. Do you experience migraines with an aura or prodrome?	Migraine (72)	0	0	0	1	0	0	1
Q54. Have you been diagnosed with depression?	Depression (60)	1	1	1	1	0	0	4
FAMILY HISTORY								
Q55. Do you have a family history of polycystic kidney disease?	Family History (66)	0	0	0	0	2	1	3
Q56. Do you have a family history of any of these conditions: ischemic stroke, carotid stenosis or other blocked arteries, heart attack, or angina?	Family History (66)	2	1	1	1	0	0	5
Q57. Do you have a family history of hypertension?	Family History (66)	0	0	1	0	0	1	2
Q58. Do you have a family history of sickle-cell disease or any of the blood diseases listed in question 49?	Family History (66)	0	0	0	2	0	0	2

Question	Heading	ISCHEMIC				HEMORRHAGIC		Overall
		A	B	C	D	E	F	
FAMILY HISTORY								
Q59. Do you have a family history of blood clots in the legs?	Family History (66)	0	0	0	1	0	0	1
Q60. Do you have a family history of intracranial aneurysms, vascular malformations in the brain, or brain hemorrhage?	Family History (66)	0	0	0	0	2	2	4

* Oral contraceptives, hormone replacement therapy, and antiplatelet agents have positive and negative effects on stroke risk. Because we designed the assessment to deal only with factors that increase risk, the benefits of these medications do not come into play in the overall risk index. The overall risk index for oral contraceptives/hormone replacement therapy is closer to 1 than 3, because estrogen conveys a protective effect against atherosclerotic stroke (column A) that would be equivalent to –2 if the assessment used negative numbers. Likewise, the overall stroke index for antiplatelet drugs is closer to –1, because these drugs convey a protective effect of approximately –1 against atherosclerotic (column A), cardioembolic (column B), and other (column D) ischemic stroke. Do not be alarmed if your doctor has prescribed antiplatelet agents for you.

HOW TO SCORE THE ASSESSMENT

You now have a list of your personal risk factors for stroke, followed by a series of numbers. To find out how these risk factors affect your stroke risk, add each column vertically. This gives you six or seven individual scores: one for each stroke subtype and one for the overall risk index, if you recorded those numbers. If you did not record the numbers of the overall risk index, add the totals of the six subtype scores together to determine your overall risk index. Use these totals to determine if you are at low, moderate, or high risk of having a certain type or types of stroke or of having any stroke, according to the following scoring system.

ISCHEMIC STROKE

Atherosclerotic (A)	less than 11	Low
	11–22	Moderate
	23 and above	High
Cardioembolic (B)	less than 11	Low
	11–22	Moderate
	23 and above	High
Lacunar (C)	Less than 10	Low
	10–20	Moderate
	21 and above	High
Other Ischemic (D)	Less than 8	Low
	8–16	Moderate
	17 and above	High

HEMORRHAGIC STROKE

Subarachnoid Hemorrhage (E)	Less than 8	Low
	8–16	Moderate
	17 and above	High
Intracerebral Hemorrhage (F)	Less than 9	Low
	9–18	Moderate
	19 and above	High
Overall Risk Index	Less than 45	Low
	45–90	Moderate
	91 and above	High

UNDERSTANDING YOUR SCORES

You now know what your stroke risk factors are, your degree of risk, and the type of stroke to which you are most prone. This gives you valuable insight into the actions you need to take to prevent stroke. If you're at moderate or high risk for stroke in general or for one or more of the various subtypes, don't panic. You can do plenty to address the risk factors that put you at risk—and take other steps to reduce your risk in those categories.

You can determine how your future actions will affect your stroke risk by recalculating your score after removing the stroke risk factors over which you have control. If you have hypertension, diabetes, or high cholesterol, but have the condition under control, for example, recalculate your score after removing the scores those conditions convey. Because these conditions themselves carry some risk, it is unlikely that your real risk will be exactly zero, but if you have them under tight control, you should be able to reduce most of the risk that accompanies them.

If you're at low risk, you should still consider taking steps to reduce your risk. After all, you will age. You can find out how age will ultimately affect your risk by recalculating your scores using the scores for an older age category.

Let me walk you through an example.

Bob is a seventy-two-year-old Caucasian man. He has mild hypertension and diabetes mellitus, both of which are under control. He does not drink alcohol, he eats a high-cholesterol, high-fat diet, and he has a family history of hypertension.

Here's what Bob's quiz paper will look like:

Factor	A Athero	B Cardiac	C Lacunar	D Other	E SAH	F ICA
Q1 Gender	2	2	1	1	0	1
Q4 Race	2	1	1	0	0	0
Q8 Age	4	3	3	2	2	3
Q15 Alcohol	2	0	0	0	0	0
Q17 Diet	3	1	1	0	0	0
Q44 Hypertension	5	3	6	3	0	5
Q46 Diabetes Mellitus	5	0	2	0	0	0
Q57 Family History	0	0	1	0	0	1
Totals	23	10	15	6	2	10 = 66

Overall Risk Index 66

As you can see from the numbers, Bob is at moderate risk of having a stroke (total stroke index 66). He is most prone to the atherosclerotic ischemic subtype, for which he is at high risk. This is where he needs to focus most of his attention regarding prevention strategies. Although he is at low risk for the cardioembolic subtype, he is approaching moderate risk. He is at moderate risk for the lacunar subtype, low risk for the other ischemic subtype, low risk for subarachnoid hemorrhage, and moderate risk for intracerebral hemorrhage.

In three years, when Bob turns seventy-five, his risk will jump substantially. He'll add four points to his atherosclerotic risk, two points to his cardioembolic risk, two points to his lacunar risk, one point each to his other ischemic and subarachnoid hemorrhage risk, and three points to his intracerebral hemorrhage risk. This will put him into the high-risk category for cardioembolic stroke and raise his overall risk index to 79.

But Bob has both his hypertension and diabetes under control. If we calculate his score again, removing those risk factors, we'll see that things aren't as bad for Bob as they appear to be.

Factor	Athero	Cardiac	Lacunar	Other	SAH	ICA
Q1 Gender	2	2	1	1	0	1
Q4 Race	2	1	1	0	0	0
Q8 Age	4	3	3	2	2	3
Q15 Alcohol	2	0	0	0	0	0
Q17 Diet	3	1	1	0	0	0
Q57 Family History	0	0	1	0	0	1
Totals	13	7	7	3	2	5 = 37

Overall Risk Index 37

You can see how important it is for Bob to maintain control over his hypertension and diabetes. By doing so, he reduces his overall stroke risk (overall risk index from 66 to 37), moving it into the low category. Although he's still at moderate risk of having an atherosclerotic ischemic stroke, he is at low risk for every other subtype. If you look at the risk factors that place Bob at high risk for atherosclerotic stroke, you'll see that he has room to reduce his risk further. Diet, for instance, can be controlled. If Bob can successfully change his diet, he can reduce his atherosclerotic ischemic stroke risk into the low category.

WHAT TO DO NEXT

Bob's case illustrates that stroke risk is something over which we have some control. We simply have to take action. You have the tools you need to get started: You know your risk factors, your degree of risk, and the type(s) of stroke to which you are most susceptible. Your first step in addressing your risk factors and reducing your risk is to educate yourself.

Start by going back to chapter 2, "The Anatomy of a Brain Attack," to refresh your memory about the subtype(s) of stroke for which you are at risk. The subtypes are described on pages 18–28. You also need to learn about the factors that place you at risk. Read the discussions of the risk factors that pertain to you in this chapter, if you have not done so already. You may also want to read about other risk factors that may be of interest to you. These factors (referred to in the heading category in the quiz) are discussed in alphabetical order in the pages that follow. The page numbers are listed in the quiz you just completed.

When you have read about the risk factors that interest you, it's time for you to develop your own personal prescription for stroke prevention. If you are at moderate or high risk, start by turning to chapter 4, "Preventing Your Stroke." There you will find descriptions of the various treatment options for each of the modifiable risk factors covered in this chapter, under the same headings and, again, in alphabetical order. (There are no entries for such nonmodifiable risk factors as age, gender, race, and family history.) Your goal is to reduce or control your risk factors, then proceed to the maintenance program described in chapter 5, "The Stroke-Free for Life Prevention Plan." If you are already at low risk, proceed directly to chapter 5 to learn how to keep your risk low. Regardless of your risk, be sure to consult with your doctor in designing your plan.

UNDERSTANDING AND EVALUATING RISK FACTORS

It should come as no surprise to you that the risk factors for stroke are often directly related to the direct causes of stroke. Research has determined conclusively that conditions like atherosclerosis, hypertension, diabetes mellitus, various heart and blood diseases, intracranial aneurysms, and vascular malformations in the brain increase stroke risk. As with many other conditions, age, gender, and race also play a role. At least one lifestyle factor—smoking—has also been conclusively linked to stroke risk. These factors account for a large number of the questions included in the stroke assessment. But what about the other questions?

Medical research is ongoing, because the more we learn about a disease or condition, the more we question. Once we discover the causes of a disease, we want to learn how to prevent it. Another reason for the persistence of research is that each study offers only one piece of the picture—pieces that may conflict or may appear to conflict. For this reason, multiple studies are needed to develop a widely accepted body of knowledge about a particular subject. After years of research, it is widely accepted that the factors I have mentioned above increase stroke risk. Research continues into other factors that may play a role in increasing the risk of stroke.

Although this research has not yet produced results that can be considered conclusive—indeed, research on some of these factors has been conflicting—I believe enough information exists about some of these risk factors—family history, dietary cholesterol and fat, alcohol, fruit and vegetable consumption, exercise, body mass index, oral contraceptives and hormone replacement therapy, such psychological factors as stress and depression, and activities that rapidly raise blood pressure—to include them in the assessment. I attribute the conflicting reports to the fact that most studies look at a risk factor's effect on overall stroke risk rather than on the risk of a certain type of stroke. More detailed study will determine if I'm right. Since we have complete or partial control over many of these factors, I believe it is worthwhile to address them before all the results are in.

To make it easy to find the risk factor or factors that pertain to you, I discuss them in alphabetical order. Here is the order in which they are discussed. The terms are those in the heading column in the questionnaire.

Age

Age is something over which we have no control, although no doubt we've all sometimes wished otherwise. Aging increases the risk of many medical conditions, and stroke is no exception. The vast majority of ischemic strokes—about 75 percent—occur in people who are sixty-five or older. Aging doesn't actually cause ischemic stroke, but because so many risk factors for the disease are chronic or ongoing, because our actions can figuratively speed up the clock, time can take its toll on the cerebrovascular system. Age also has an effect on both types of hemorrhagic stroke—subarachnoid hemorrhage and intracerebral hemorrhage.

Aging begins to affect stroke risk at about forty-five. The risk then increases with each decade. Because there is relatively little you can do about this risk factor, if you are older, it is in your best interest for you to take action to reduce any risk factors you *can* control—or to do what you can to prevent risk factors from developing. If everyone worked toward preventing risk factors at a younger age, age would not have the effect it now does.

Alcohol

You've probably read or heard that alcohol can be both good and bad for the heart. I believe the same is true for the brain, although for different reasons, and studies bear me out. Some studies indicate that light to moderate alcohol consumption is protective; others indicate that heavy alcohol consumption may increase not only the risk of stroke but also the risk of death from stroke.

Clearly, the benefit or risk posed by alcohol is in large part related to the amount. Alcohol abuse or binge drinking is unhealthy. It increases blood pressure and has variable effects on blood clotting. It can also cause cardiomyopathy (disease of the heart muscle) and, possibly, atrial fibrillation (a common heart rhythm disorder). All of these factors have the potential to increase ischemic stroke risk. In fact, Finnish researchers reported in 1999 that people who drank between thirteen and twenty-five drinks a week were four times more likely to have a stroke than those who didn't drink.

The conflicting findings about alcohol are also likely related to stroke type. The Finnish study, for example, found that heavy alcohol intake increased the rate of cardioembolic stroke, the type caused by clots that originate in the heart. Other studies indicate that alcohol may lower the risk of certain types of ischemic stroke—particularly atherosclerotic stroke— and increase or have no effect on the risk of hemorrhagic stroke. A recent study of 22,000 male doctors, for example, found that those who had at least one drink a week had a 21 percent lower risk of stroke in general and a 23 percent lower risk of ischemic stroke. Alcohol consumption had no effect, positive or negative, on the risk of hemorrhagic stroke. Still other studies indicate that alcohol contributes to a higher rate of subarachnoid hemorrhage and, possibly, intracerebral hemorrhage.

Excessive drinking or binge drinking is unhealthy by all accounts, particularly if you have other risk factors for hemorrhagic stroke. Mild to moderate drinking may be protective if you have atherosclerosis or are prone to the atherosclerotic subtype of ischemic stroke. I don't want to encourage anyone with an alcohol problem to start drinking. If you're not a drinker and you have one or more of the other risk factors for atherosclerotic stroke, you may be missing out on an opportunity to reduce your risk. You might want to consider having an occasional drink—say, a glass of wine with dinner or a cold beer on a hot day. Just don't overdo it. There's a fine line between when alcohol reduces risk and when it increases risk. That line is drawn in large part by amount. To get a protective effect from alcohol, you need to drink in moderation. Moderate drinking generally means no more than two drinks per day.

Anticoagulants

Anticoagulants, known commonly as blood thinners, are crucial to the treatment of ischemic stroke, certain heart conditions, and other blood clotting disorders. These potentially lifesaving drugs do have the ability to trigger bleeding in the brain and cause hemorrhagic stroke. The most commonly prescribed anticoagulant drug is warfarin (Coumadin, Panwarfin). Other anticoagulant drugs, given by injection, include heparin and heparinoids. Thrombolytic, or clot-busting, agents like streptokinase, urokinase, and tissue plasminogen activator (tPA), which are generally given to treat acute heart attack or ischemic stroke, also have the potential to trigger hemorrhage.

You should know what medications you are taking. Ask your doctor or pharmacist if you don't. Generally speaking, you may be taking an anticoagulant if you have a mechanical heart valve, a history of blood clots (in the veins of the leg, for example), a heart condition like atrial fibrillation, cardiomyopathy, or recent heart attack, or if you have had a transient ischemic attack and have been diagnosed with underlying blockages in arteries that are not appropriate for surgery.

Antiplatelet Agents

Aspirin and other antiplatelet agents have a mild blood-thinning effect and, thus, may increase hemorrhagic stroke risk. The risk these drugs convey is not nearly as great as that posed by anticoagulant medications, but it is present nonetheless. It's hard to quantify this risk in research because aspirin use is often sporadic and not indicated in many people's medical records. Although your doctor may know—and in fact may have recommended— that you take aspirin regularly if you have ischemic heart disease, he or she is unlikely to know that you generally take an aspirin two or three times a week for headaches or other pains.

You, however, should know what medications you are taking. Ask your doctor or pharmacist if you don't. You may be taking an antiplatelet agent such as aspirin, dipyridamole (Persantine), a combination of aspirin and dipyridamole (Aggrenox), clopidogrel (Plavix), or ticlopidine (Ticlid) if you have been diagnosed with atherosclerosis or ischemic heart disease. You may also be taking aspirin for any of a number of reasons. If your doctor has recommended that you take antiplatelet agents, don't be alarmed by the apparent risk conveyed by the quiz. Although these medications convey a slight risk of hemorrhagic stroke, they offer protection against ischemic stroke. In general, they are likely to decrease overall stroke risk.

Arteritis

Arteritis is an inflammation of the walls of the arteries. This inflammation can lead to swelling that can obstruct the arteries. If it obstructs the arteries that supply the brain, it can cause ischemic stroke. The condition also conveys a slightly increased risk of intracerebral and subarachnoid hemorrhage. This inflammation may be caused by certain diseases, including systemic lupus erythematosus and Behçet's disease, by other abnormalities, or by such infectious diseases as meningitis, syphilis, malaria, herpes zoster, or trichinosis. The symptoms and diagnosis depend in large part upon the underlying cause.

Artery Blockage or Narrowing (Stenosis)

If you've been diagnosed with a blockage or narrowing in one of the arteries in your neck (the carotid or vertebral arteries) or one of the arteries in your head that supplies blood to the brain, you probably have atherosclerosis and, thus, are at risk of having an atherosclerotic ischemic stroke and, to a lesser extent, cardioembolic ischemic stroke. (In rare cases, blockages can be caused by other conditions, including trauma and fibromuscular disease. Blockages caused by these conditions do not increase the risk of atherosclerotic ischemic stroke.) Atherosclerosis, a buildup of fatty deposits known as plaque along the inside of artery walls, contributes to stroke in two ways. As it progresses, atherosclerosis narrows arteries, making it easier for a clot to become lodged within them. In some cases, the narrowing itself partially or completely blocks the arteries. This narrowing is known as *stenosis*. In addition, the plaque attracts blood products and, thus, can generate clots.

Carotid artery stenosis is an important cause of transient ischemic attack and minor ischemic stroke, which essentially are its primary symptoms. Another possible sign is a carotid bruit, a "swishing" sound (*bruit* is French for "sound") in the artery that can be detected by a stethoscope. If your doctor has detected such a sound in your neck, he or she will likely suggest a series of exams and tests to determine the extent of the blockage. The exams will likely include a neurologic exam, a series of observations, questions, and tasks designed to determine if your muscles, reflexes, and cognitive skills are functioning correctly; and an examination of your eye with an ophthalmoscope. The tests will probably also include at least one test designed to evaluate the carotid artery itself. These tests could include carotid ultrasound, which produces an image by bouncing sound waves off the carotid artery and other structures in the neck, and ocular pneumoplethysmography, which measures the systolic blood pressure in the ophthalmic arteries, which supply the eye with blood. These arteries branch off from the carotid arteries and, thus, can reflect blockages in those arteries.

Doctors measure blockages of the carotid arteries using percentages that reflect the arteries' diameter. Generally speaking, the risk is higher and treatment is more often suggested in cases where the reduction is 60 percent or more in the absence of associated symptoms.

Atrial Fibrillation

Atrial fibrillation is a common arrhythmia, or heart rhythm disorder. In atrial fibrillation, the walls of the heart's atria, or upper chambers, beat rapidly, which causes an irregular rhythm. This irregular rhythm can occur periodically or continually. When it occurs periodically, we refer to it as *intermittent atrial fibrillation;* when it occurs continually, we refer to it as *persistent atrial fibrillation.* In either case, the symptoms may include palpitations (pounding or racing heartbeat), chest pain, shortness of breath, fatigue, and light-headedness. Your doctor may diagnose atrial fibrillation when he or she investigates the cause of your symptoms or may uncover it in the results of a routine electrocardiogram. The electrocardiogram, which clearly shows the irregular, rapid beating of the heart, is the test most often used to diagnose the condition. Unfortunately, the condition is often diagnosed only after it has caused a transient ischemic attack or ischemic stroke.

Atrial fibrillation can weaken the heart muscle and can occasionally lead to congestive heart failure. It can also present a serious problem in its own right. Since the atria are pumping ineffectively, blood can pool within them and form a clot, and clots from the heart can travel to the arteries that supply the brain. Atrial fibrillation may also contribute to ischemic stroke in a more subtle way. Ongoing research at Mayo Clinic indicates that irregular heart rhythm may be a marker of an underlying problem with endothelial tissue, tissue that lines the heart, blood vessels, lymph vessels, and certain body cavities. This endothelial dysfunction may predispose a person to atrial fibrillation, congestive heart failure, and, possibly, atherosclerosis and hypertension, making it an independent risk factor for ischemic stroke.

Approximately 15 percent of people with atrial fibrillation experience ischemic strokes. Atrial fibrillation is a leading risk factor and certainly one of the most important cardiac risk factors, but the actual risk it conveys varies based on type, duration, and the presence of other risk factors. Generally speaking, people with intermittent atrial fibrillation are at a slightly higher risk of ischemic stroke than are people with persistent atrial fibrillation. The starting and stopping of the irregular heartbeat makes blood more likely to pool in the atria and form a clot. The duration of the condition also affects risk. The risk is generally at its highest if the condition has recently been diagnosed. This is because diagnosis so often follows an event, for example, TIA, that is a strong indicator of a future ischemic stroke. This does not mean that you're at low risk if you've had the condition for some time. Risk accumulates with time. Although your risk from year to year may be fairly similar, the slight increases from year to year do add up. The risk also increases when atrial fibrillation is accompanied by such other risk factors as hypertension, congestive heart failure, a history of blood clots, mitral or aortic heart valve disease, and an enlarged left atrium.

Bleeding Disorders

Bleeding disorders like hemophilia, an inherited deficiency of certain blood clotting factors, thrombocytopenia, a shortage of blood platelets, and other conditions that affect blood's ability to clot properly can lead to hemorrhages almost anywhere in the body, including the head. It is therefore no surprise that these conditions would be associated with an increased risk of hemorrhagic stroke. They can also make it more difficult to manage hemorrhagic stroke caused by another factor. Their effect is less pronounced if they are controlled by medications or other means.

Body Mass Index

Body mass index, or BMI, is a measurement that takes into account both height and weight. This measurement, which is obtained by dividing metric weight by metric height squared, is considered a more accurate way to determine healthy weight than the height-weight charts of old. You can find your BMI by referring to the chart in Appendix A. A BMI of 25 or greater is considered overweight; a BMI less than 19 is considered underweight.

Maintaining a healthy weight can provide some protection against stroke. Although being overweight is not an independent risk factor for stroke, overall there is a tendency for people with increased BMI to have a greater risk of ischemic stroke and intracerebral hemorrhage. Being overweight places you at risk for high blood pressure, ischemic heart disease, diabetes mellitus, and high total and LDL cholesterol levels. It can also increase triglyceride levels and lower HDL cholesterol levels. All of these factors can increase your risk of ischemic stroke. High blood pressure can also increase your risk of intracerebral hemorrhage.

Being underweight may pose problems of its own. There is some evidence that underweight individuals are at increased risk for subarachnoid hemorrhage.

Cardiomyopathy

Cardiomyopathy is a disease of the heart muscle that affects the heart's ability to pump. It comes in several varieties, including *dilated,* in which the muscle weakens and the heart chambers dilate, or enlarge; *hypertrophic,* in which the muscle becomes extremely thick; and *restrictive,* in which the muscle stiffens and the heart cannot adequately fill with blood. In many cases, the cause of these problems remains unknown. In other cases, they can be linked to such culprits as infection; exposure to drugs, alcohol, and other toxins; myocarditis, or inflammation of the myocardium, or heart muscle; ischemic heart disease (coronary-artery disease); long-term chronic hypertension; and such genetically determined conditions as hemochromatosis, an inherited disorder in which the body does not metabolize iron effectively.

Cardiomyopathy can be a serious condition in its own right. It can also lead to other problems, including irregular heart rhythms and congestive heart failure. And it increases the risk of the cardioembolic subtype of ischemic stroke. The symptoms of cardiomyopathy vary based on the type but include shortness of breath, swelling in the legs, abdominal and/or chest pain, and, occasionally, loss of consciousness with exertion. These symptoms, accompanied by a physical exam and a medical history, can lead your doctor to the diagnosis. The diagnosis can be confirmed with one or more tests, including electrocardiography (ECG or EKG), which records the heart's electrical impulses, and echocardiography, a type of ultrasound that can measure the contraction of the left ventricle. If your doctor cannot distinguish whether your symptoms are caused by a blocked coronary artery, he or she may recommend cardiac catheterization or a stress test.

Cholesterol and Triglyceride Levels

High levels of cholesterol in the blood are known to accelerate the development of atherosclerosis, a risk factor for ischemic stroke and certain forms of heart disease. It would seem, then, that reducing blood cholesterol levels would lower the risk of stroke, but studies on the subject have been inconclusive. In many studies high blood cholesterol has not appeared to increase the risk of stroke, but these studies have not examined the various subtypes of ischemic stroke—and many have not even examined ischemic versus hemorrhagic stroke. I strongly suspect that a high blood cholesterol level—a level above 200 mg/dL—substantially increases the risk of atherosclerotic ischemic stroke and likely conveys a slight increase in the risk for cardioembolic and lacunar ischemic stroke.

Cholesterol is produced by the liver from dietary fats. It is also present in certain foods, including meat, eggs, and dairy products. A person's blood cholesterol level is determined in large part by his or her dietary intake of fat and cholesterol, although there is also a genetic component. An Australian population study found that people who ate meat more than four times a week were at an increased risk of stroke, while those who used reduced-fat milk were at a lower risk, which supports the theory that dietary cholesterol and fat are risk factors for ischemic stroke. I believe these dietary factors are particularly important for people with such other risk factors for atherosclerotic stroke as family history, ischemic heart disease, and TIA.

Generally speaking, a total blood cholesterol level of 200 mg/dL or above is considered high and should be viewed as a red flag. This means that you're taking in too much cholesterol and saturated fat from your diet, and/or your body is producing too much cholesterol. Although this waxlike substance is essential for health, excess amounts in the blood tend to stick to the artery walls, resulting in the buildup of atherosclerotic deposits. The primary culprit is a type of cholesterol known as low-density lipoprotein, or LDL. Triglycerides, another type of blood fat, are also unhealthy. To reduce your risk of developing atherosclerosis or to slow the progress of atherosclerotic buildup, your LDL number should be below 130 mg/dL and your triglyceride number below 200 mg/dL. Another type of cholesterol, high-density lipoprotein, or HDL, helps escort LDL out of the body, which lowers total cholesterol levels. A healthy HDL level is 45 mg/dL or higher. I have found that the ideal numbers to aspire to are 150 mg/dL for total cholesterol, below 100 mg/dL for LDL, and above 50 mg/dL for HDL.

To find out your cholesterol levels, you must take a complete lipid profile. This is a simple blood test, often included as part of a complete physical exam, that involves giving several tubes of blood from a vein in your arm. The blood is then analyzed to measure levels of total cholesterol, LDL, HDL, and triglycerides.

Clot in the Heart

Many of the conditions covered in this section pose risk because they can generate the formation of a clot in the heart. It makes sense, then, that a clot that has already formed in your heart is a risk factor for cardioembolic stroke. If you've been diagnosed with a clot in your heart, there's the chance that the clot can become dislodged and travel to one of the arteries that supplies blood to the brain.

If you've been diagnosed with a clot in the heart, you probably know it: your doctor probably initiated treatment shortly after the diagnosis was made, and chances are good that you've also been diagnosed with one of the conditions that leads to clot formation, for example atrial fibrillation, congestive heart failure, valvular heart disease, or a recent heart attack. A clot in the heart can be diagnosed using echocardiography or another form of ultrasound or angiography.

Congenital Heart Defects

Congenital heart defects are heart defects that are present at birth. They range from abnormalities of the blood vessels or valves to defects in the partitions that divide the chambers of the heart to problematic connections between the blood vessels and the heart. They may be caused by inherited genetic problems, environmental exposure during development, or a combination, and they range in severity from minor to life-threatening. Although many of these problems can now be detected by ultrasound in the womb, in other cases, they may not become apparent at all—or until they cause a problem later in life. Some valvular defects, for example, may not become apparent until the passage of time takes its effect on the valve and symptoms of valvular disease appear. Congenital heart defects can increase the risk of the cardioembolic subtype of ischemic stroke.

Congestive Heart Failure

Congestive heart failure, known simply as heart failure, is the term used to describe symptoms and diseases that affect the heart's ability to pump blood effectively. It does not mean, as the term seems to imply, that the heart simply stops working. Congestive heart failure, which affects more than 4 million Americans, can be caused by any of a number of heart conditions, including valvular heart disease, congenital heart disease, long-term hypertension, and the damage caused by a heart attack. When these or other conditions weaken the heart or affect its ability to supply blood throughout the body, the result is heart failure and increased risk of ischemic stroke.

Symptoms of heart failure range from mild shortness of breath during physical activity to shortness of breath and fatigue even when resting. Other symptoms include swelling in the legs and feet and, in severe cases, irregular heart rhythms, palpitations (pounding or racing heart), fainting, and a blue tint to the skin. These symptoms, coupled with a history of the types of heart disease that can lead to congestive heart failure, may indicate the condition. To confirm the diagnosis, your doctor may suggest one or more tests, including a nuclear scan, which measures the size of the heart chambers and evaluates the chambers' pumping ability; echocardiography, which can show heart and chamber size and function, pumping strength, and damage to the heart muscle; and angiography.

Depression

Depression may increase the risk of ischemic stroke. Recent studies have found that people who are depressed are more likely to die of heart problems, to die after a heart attack, and to develop ischemic heart disease. Depression appears to affect the blood and the blood vessels and may promote the development of clots. This clearly could have an effect on ischemic stroke risk. Several studies have found that ischemic stroke rates are higher in people who have symptoms of depression, though other studies have produced conflicting results. None of the studies specified stroke risk by subtype. I believe that depression may increase the risk of all types of ischemic stroke and possibly of intracerebral hemorrhage, although this is less likely. We are currently conducting a study to evaluate these hypotheses.

Depression is generally diagnosed based on the symptoms, which include:

- depressed mood most of the day, nearly every day
- diminished interest in all, or most, activities most of the day, nearly every day
- unintentional weight loss or gain
- insomnia or hypersomnia (sleeping too much) nearly every day
- abnormal speeding up or slowing down of activities and mental processes nearly every day
- fatigue or lack of energy nearly every day
- feelings of worthlessness or guilt
- reduced ability to concentrate or think nearly every day
- recurrent thoughts of death

Generally speaking, at least five of these symptoms must be present within the same two-week period for your doctor to diagnose you with major depressive disorder. An occasional blue feeling every now and then is perfectly normal and does not indicate a problem. You may notice these symptoms yourself or a friend or relative may notice them. Your doctor will likely detect them by asking you to fill out a questionnaire and by talking with you and, perhaps, your family or friends. Your doctor might also give you a mental status exam. You may undergo laboratory or other diagnostic tests if you have other symptoms or your doctor needs to rule out another condition that may cause symptoms similar to those of depression.

Diabetes Mellitus

Diabetes mellitus is a metabolic disorder in which the body cannot convert carbohydrates into energy. Specifically, it is an inability to produce or use the hormone insulin, which results in high levels of sugar in the blood. Diabetes increases the risk of ischemic stroke, particularly the atherosclerotic subtype and, to a lesser extent, the lacunar subtype. The disease often appears in conjunction with other risk factors, including hypertension and heart disease, but studies indicate that it is a risk factor in and of itself. We don't know exactly how diabetes increases stroke risk. We do know that the disease affects and changes blood vessels, particularly smaller blood vessels. The high blood sugar it causes may also contribute to stroke risk and severity. Some studies have found that when people with high blood sugar experience ischemic stroke, they suffer more damage than people with normal blood sugar.

An estimated 16 million Americans have diabetes mellitus, but approximately 6 million of these people do not know they have the disease. This is partly because diabetes does not always produce symptoms, and the symptoms it does produce are not always obvious or may be symptoms of other disorders. These symptoms include frequent urination, thirst, weight loss, visual disturbances, skin disorders, itching, and pain and/or numbness of the extremities. Diagnosis may be based on the appearance of these symptoms, coupled with tests that indicate high levels of glucose, or sugar, in blood and/or urine tests. If symptoms aren't present, diagnosis is based primarily on the results of blood and/or urine tests.

Diet

When it comes to stroke risk, it's true that you are what you eat. A diet high in cholesterol or saturated fat can increase your blood cholesterol level, thereby increasing your risk of atherosclerosis and atherosclerotic ischemic stroke, and, to a lesser degree, of cardioembolic and lacunar ischemic stroke. This is because the body gets some of its cholesterol directly from diet and makes the rest, largely from the saturated fats you eat. The foods highest in cholesterol and saturated fat are such animal foods as meats, dairy products, and eggs. You can find the cholesterol and fat content of packaged foods by reading the Nutrition Facts label.

A diet low in fruits and vegetables can also increase your risk of ischemic stroke, particularly the atherosclerotic subtype and, to a lesser extent, the cardioembolic and lacunar subtypes. This is partly because people who tend to eat fewer fruits and vegetables tend to eat more foods containing cholesterol and saturated fat. Fruits and vegetables may also offer some independent protection against ischemic stroke. Although earlier studies that looked at fruit and vegetable intake produced conflicting results, Harvard School of Public Health researchers made headlines in 1999 for reporting that fruits and vegetables (excluding potatoes, soybeans, and dried beans and lentils) offer protection against ischemic stroke. Specifically, the researchers found that people who ate five to six servings a day were 31 percent less likely to have an ischemic stroke than those who ate fewer than three servings. The most potent effects were found in citrus fruits, citrus juice, green leafy vegetables, and cruciferous vegetables like broccoli, cabbage, and cauliflower. Possible sources of this apparent protective effect include potassium, folate, fiber, and dietary flavonoids. Several earlier studies have linked a potassium-rich diet to a reduced risk of ischemic stroke, particularly among men with high blood pressure.

Another dietary factor that may slightly increase your risk of stroke, particularly the lacunar subtype of ischemic stroke and intracerebral hemorrhage, is sodium, a primary ingredient of salt. A high intake of sodium can increase blood pressure in people who are sodium-sensitive. Hypertension is the primary cause of lacunar stroke and intracerebral hemorrhage. Sodium intake also slightly increases the risk of atherosclerotic ischemic stroke. You may be taking in too much sodium if you eat a lot of salty foods or processed foods that are high in sodium or if you add a lot of salt to your food. Nutrition Facts labels on processed foods indicate the amount of sodium in a product.

Diseases Linked to Intracranial Aneurysms

Although we do not yet know all the various factors that come into play in the development of intracranial aneurysms, we have found that certain medical conditions may play a role in their development. These conditions include:

polycystic kidney disease, an inherited disorder characterized by the development of cysts within the kidneys

coarctation of the aorta, a congenital heart defect in which the aorta, the body's primary artery, is narrowed or constricted

Marfan's syndrome, an inherited condition characterized by elongated bones and muscular problems along with abnormalities of the cardiovascular system

Ehlers-Danlos syndrome, a hereditary condition that affects the connective tissue, including the skin and joints

fibromuscular dysplasia, a noninflammatory disease that often affects the internal carotid arteries

pseudoxanthoma elasticum, an inherited disorder characterized by the degeneration of tissue and vascular disturbances

moyamoya disease, a condition often characterized by a network of small blood vessels that replace the normal blood vessels around the base of the brain because of narrowing or blockage in large arteries supplying the brain

neurofibromatosis, an inherited condition characterized by fibrous tumors on nerve tissue, including the skin; birth marks; and other developmental problems of the bones and muscles

arteriovenous malformations (see vascular malformation section, page 83)

certain **tumors** involving the pituitary gland

If you have been diagnosed with any of these conditions, you may be at increased risk of developing an intracranial aneurysm, which can put you at increased risk of subarachnoid and intracerebral hemorrhage. This does not mean that you will develop an aneurysm.

Disorders That Cause Increased Clotting

A variety of blood disorders can increase the risk of ischemic stroke by thickening the blood or making it more likely to clot. These conditions include:

polycythemia, in which the blood contains an elevated level of red blood cells

thrombocythemia, in which the blood contains an elevated number of platelets

thrombocytopenic purpura, in which the blood contains a decreased number of platelets

dysproteinemia, in which the protein content of the blood is abnormal

antiphospholipid antibody syndrome, in which the blood contains antibodies that affect blood clotting

leukemia, a cancer of the white blood cells

disseminated intravascular coagulation, a condition in which tissue damage from trauma, burns, or infection causes the blood to release clotting agents.

Generally, these conditions are detected with blood tests.

Endocarditis

Endocarditis is an inflammation of the endocardium, the tissue that makes up the internal lining of the heart and the valves. Although it has several causes, including links to cancer and systemic lupus erythematosus, its most common cause is infection, usually of the heart valves. The infection itself can trigger the development of blood clots and, indeed, it does so in about 20 percent of people with infective endocarditis. In addition, endocarditis often causes valvular damage, especially in people whose heart valves are already damaged or diseased. The condition is also associated with the development of mycotic intracranial aneurysms, which increase the risk of subarachnoid hemorrhage.

People with defective or diseased heart valves and people with artificial heart valves are at increased risk of developing endocarditis. Your doctor may diagnose infective endocarditis based on symptoms, including symptoms of infection like fever, and on the results of echocardiography, which can show infected tissue on a heart valve.

Exercise

You no doubt know that exercise is good for you and that being a couch potato is unhealthy. Study after study indicates the benefits of exercise: It can prevent or reverse obesity and, in turn, help prevent or control blood pressure, diabetes, and high cholesterol. It can also have a positive effect on the heart, preventing ischemic heart disease, increasing the heart's ability to pump, and decreasing resting heart rate. Exercise helps decrease blood glucose, or sugar, it's a natural stress reliever, and it can help alleviate the symptoms of depression. Because of these benefits, regular exercise helps prevent all types of ischemic stroke as well as intracerebral hemorrhage. All told, regular exercise three or four times a week has been shown to reduce the risk of early death from all causes by about 70 percent.

The studies look at the benefits of exercising rather than the effects of being sedentary, but it's clear that a person with a sedentary lifestyle is not reaping the benefits of exercise and, as such, is increasing his or her risk.

Family History

Your family history helps define who you are. It also helps define your health. Your parents pass on their genes as well as their advice and values. We've known for centuries that certain diseases, like hemophilia, are passed from one generation to another. We've also known that other diseases, like cancer and ischemic heart disease, tend to be more common in some families than in others. This appears to be true of stroke. Some studies suggest that if your parents had a stroke, you are at an increased risk of having a stroke. If you think about it, it makes sense. Several stroke risk factors, including hypertension, diabetes, atherosclerosis, and ischemic heart disease, tend to run in families. Recent research indicates that there may be a genetic component to these risk factors. Genetics also play a role in the development of intracranial aneurysms. As research continues, I believe we will identify genes that confer susceptibility to these risk factors and, perhaps, to the various subtypes of stroke themselves.

Currently, we believe that your family medical history may confer a slightly increased risk of ischemic stroke if it includes such atherosclerotic diseases as heart attack, angina, a blockage of the carotid, or coronary arteries, or a blockage of a leg artery, or sickle-cell disease. There may be a slightly increased risk of both ischemic and hemorrhagic stroke if your history includes hypertension. And a slightly increased risk of hemorrhagic stroke may be presumed if your history includes intracranial aneurysms or polycystic kidney disease. Approximately 10 to 15 percent of people who are diagnosed with intracranial aneurysms have a family history of the balloonings. This means that an inherited predisposition is likely involved in the development of intracranial aneurysms, the leading cause of subarachnoid hemorrhage. There is also a hereditary component to polycystic kidney disease, which has been linked to intracranial aneurysms.

If any of these conditions run in your family, you may be at increased risk of developing them yourself. This does not necessarily mean that you will develop them.

Gender

In this battle of the sexes, the guys are the overall losers. Men are more likely to have an ischemic stroke than are women. They are also more likely to have an intracerebral hemorrhage. This does not mean that ischemic stroke and intracerebral hemorrhage do not affect women, but all other things being equal, men are generally at greater risk. We are not exactly sure why this is so. Men are more likely to have ischemic heart disease (you may have heard it referred to as coronary-artery disease) and high blood pressure than are women. They are more likely to smoke, eat a high-fat, high-cholesterol diet, and have a type A personality. No doubt, these factors are part of the equation. I suspect that hormonal differences may also play a role.

Women are at higher risk of subarachnoid hemorrhage than are men. This is probably related to the fact that women are three times more likely than men to develop unruptured intracranial aneurysms.

Hypertension

Hypertension, or high blood pressure, is an underlying cause of ischemic and hemorrhagic stroke. Consequently, it is also a risk factor—particularly for lacunar infarction and intracerebral hemorrhage and, to a lesser extent, for the atherosclerotic and other ischemic stroke subtypes. Hypertension, which generally produces no symptoms, can weaken the small blood vessels in the brain and cause them to deteriorate. It also can affect the heart's ability to function, and it often appears in conjunction with atherosclerosis.

Borderline hypertension, a level of 140–159/90–94 mm Hg, increases ischemic stroke risk slightly. Definite hypertension, a level above 160/95 mm Hg, increases ischemic stroke risk about twofold. Moderate to severe hypertension, a level above 180/105 mm Hg, or hypertension associated with left ventricular hypertrophy (enlargement of the heart's left ventricle), confers an even greater risk.

Chronic hypertension is also the leading cause of intracerebral hemorrhage in the population. Surprisingly, it does not seem to increase the risk of subarachnoid hemorrhage, nor does it seem to cause the development or rupture of intracranial aneurysms.

In order to be diagnosed with hypertension, you must have your blood pressure taken on more than one occasion, because blood pressure fluctuates throughout the day. Hypertension is known as the silent killer, because it rarely exhibits symptoms. Chances are good that your blood pressure is monitored somewhat regularly. Your doctor or nurse probably takes your blood pressure whenever you have a physical exam or an office visit. You can get your blood pressure checked at pharmacies, malls, and health fairs, and you can buy a blood pressure monitoring device to monitor your blood pressure at home.

Here's what the procedure entails. A cuff is placed around your arm (or, in the case of a machine like those in many pharmacies, you place your arm into a cuff). The cuff is inflated, which temporarily closes the arteries in your arm. As the pressure is gradually released, the doctor, nurse, machine—or you, if you're taking your own reading—listens to your pulse using a stethoscope placed over an artery in your arm. The point at which the first beat is heard is the systolic blood pressure (the top number in a blood pressure reading); the point at which the pulse disappears is the diastolic (or bottom) reading. A gauge on the blood pressure monitoring device provides the actual numbers.

Ongoing research at Mayo Clinic indicates that hypertension may actually be a marker of an underlying problem with endothelial tissue throughout the body. Endothelial tissue lines the heart, blood vessels, lymph vessels, and certain body cavities. Endothelial dysfunction is often present in hypertension, atherosclerosis, atrial fibrillation, congestive heart failure, and other heart conditions.

Fortunately, hypertension can be controlled, although there is now some question whether simply reducing blood pressure values is the optimal treatment. If research determines that hypertension is a marker for endothelial dysfunction, the focus of hypertension treatment may switch from simply reducing blood pressure values to reducing blood pressure and treating the underlying endothelial condition.

Hypokinetic/Akinetic Heart Segment

Hypokinetic/akinetic heart segment refers to impaired movement of the left ventricle of the heart (one of the lower chambers). This condition usually occurs as the result of heart attack or reduced oxygen to the heart and may lead to the formation of a clot in the immobile part of the heart, which can increase the risk of cardioembolic ischemic stroke. It is generally diagnosed with echocardiography, a form of ultrasound; angiography, X rays taken after a dye has been injected into the heart; or radionuclide ventriculography, an X ray of the heart's ventricle after it has been injected with a radioactive contrast medium.

Intermittent Claudication

Intermittent claudication is a periodic cramping of the calves that occurs especially after an extended period of walking, is relieved by rest, and can happen repeatedly. You might not think that the health of your legs has much connection to the health of your brain, but intermittent claudication is less an indicator of leg health than it is of circulatory health. It is a symptom of atherosclerosis and, as such, a risk factor for atherosclerotic stroke and, to a lesser extent, of cardioembolic ischemic stroke, because it conveys some risk of heart attack.

Intracranial Aneurysms

The typical intracranial aneurysm is a ballooning, or outpouching, of a weakened area of an arterial wall. These balloonings, like the weakened area of a tire, are prone to rupture, causing a "blowout" characterized by bleeding. The rupture of intracranial aneurysms is the leading cause of subarachnoid hemorrhage, accounting for an estimated 75 to 90 percent of all cases. Less commonly, it is a cause of intracerebral hemorrhage. Intracranial aneurysms are more common than we initially realized. Autopsy studies show that they exist in approximately 5 percent of the population at some point in life. They usually go undetected until or unless they rupture. The good news is that most intracranial aneurysms never rupture. However, their very presence is a risk factor for subarachnoid hemorrhage and often a source of considerable worry for patients.

One of the reasons most intracranial aneurysms go undetected is that they rarely exhibit any symptoms. There are situations, however, in which an intracranial aneurysm exhibits symptoms that warrant urgent attention, most notably, when the aneurysm leaks. Since leakage from an aneurysm indicates that the weakened blood vessel is in danger of imminent rupture, we refer to a leak as a *warning leak*. The symptoms of a warning leak are not unlike some of the symptoms of subarachnoid hemorrhage itself because a warning leak actually represents a very small subarachnoid hemorrhage. These symptoms include a sudden, uncharacteristic, severe headache that may or may not be accompanied by stiff neck, nausea, and vomiting; and a strong aversion to light. Other symptoms, which may reflect either a warning leak or symptoms other than rupture, include:

- double vision
- a droopy eyelid
- an inability to move the eyes in one or more directions
- a change in vision, particularly in one eye
- a dilated pupil on one side of the face
- numbness on one side of the face
- seizures

Although these symptoms do not always relate to intracranial aneurysms, if you experience them, you should seek medical attention immediately.

In most instances, intracranial aneurysms that have not ruptured are detected after a person has undergone an imaging test such as a computed tomography (CT) scan or magnetic resonance imaging (MRI) of the head for an unrelated condition or problem, or magnetic resonance angiography (MRA) or arteriography. You generally will not know if you have an intracranial aneurysm unless you have undergone such a test.

Ischemic Heart Disease

Ischemic heart disease, like ischemic stroke, is characterized by a lack of blood and oxygen. In ischemic heart disease, the deprived organ is the heart, rather than the brain. It's most often associated with atherosclerotic blockage of one of the coronary arteries (coronary-artery disease), and its most common manifestations are heart attack and the chest pain known as angina. Either of these conditions indicates ischemic heart disease—especially if your medical history and the results of a physical exam also point to that diagnosis. Your doctor may choose one or more of a number of tests to confirm the diagnosis. These tests, which are described below, range from simple blood tests to more complex tests, including electrocardiography, echocardiography, nuclear scanning, catheterization, and angiography.

Blood tests cannot actually diagnose ischemic heart disease, but they can indicate whether you have certain predisposing factors to the disease. Among the tests that may be conducted are those for blood levels of lipids, or fats, like cholesterol and triglycerides; those for blood levels of certain cardiac enzymes that may indicate damage to the heart; and those that determine the amount of oxygen circulating in your blood.

Electrocardiography measures the electrical impulses given off by the heart. You may have heard it referred to as ECG or EKG. For this test, small electrodes connected to a machine called an electrocardiograph are temporarily attached to your skin. The electrodes pick up the electrical activity of your heart, and the machine translates the findings into a graph of your heart rate and rhythm. Abnormalities of this graph, or wave, can sometimes indicate whether a heart attack has occurred or whether the heart muscle is getting enough oxygen. If your doctor suspects that your heart isn't getting enough oxygen, he or she may recommend an exercise ECG, or stress test. This test is essentially an ECG test performed before, during, and after you exercise. It is commonly performed to diagnose ischemic heart disease, because the abnormalities related to ischemia often occur during exercise.

Another test used to diagnose ischemic heart disease is echocardiography, a specialized form of ultrasound. In echocardiography, a doctor or technician waves a device called a transducer over your heart. This device sends sound waves and detects their echoes as they bounce off the surfaces of the internal structures. The echoes are fed into a machine that uses the information to generate an image of the heart. Echocardiography images can be used to measure your heart's size and shape, detect abnormalities or damage to the heart muscle, determine the heart's pumping ability, measure narrowing in heart valves, and indicate blood flow. It can be performed while you are at rest or, like electrocardiography, during and after you have exercised.

In nuclear scanning, a small amount of a radioactive substance is injected into your bloodstream and detected by special equipment that uses it to create a computer-generated image of the heart. This image can show the chamber size and pumping ability of the heart as well as the blood flow to the heart muscle and lungs. Like the ECG and echocardiography, this test can be performed either at rest or before and after exercise.

If your doctor suspects a blockage of your coronary arteries, the arteries that supply blood to the heart, he or she may suggest catheterization and/or angiography. The procedure involves inserting a thin, flexible tube known as a catheter into certain blood vessels or the heart itself. Depending on the type of catheter, it may measure the amount of oxygen in the blood or the pressure and blood flow within the heart or blood vessels. The catheter can also be used to inject a dye or other contrast agent into your arteries so that the vessels become visible on X rays. Catheterization and angiography are generally among the final tests used to diagnose ischemic heart disease because they are invasive and carry some risks, including bruising, the formation of a bulge or blockage in an artery, bleeding, localized numbness, or allergic reaction to the contrast medium.

Migraine

Migraine headaches can very mildly increase ischemic stroke risk—particularly in women who also smoke and take birth control pills. Those most at risk are those whose headaches are preceded by a prodrome, or aura—sensations of lights, sound, visual disturbances, or numbness. Fortunately, only about 10 to 20 percent of people who experience migraines experience these sensations, and only a very small percentage of them experience ischemic stroke. During these incidents, the arteries that supply part of the brain constrict in spasm, depriving certain areas of the brain of blood and oxygen—a mechanism similar to ischemic stroke.

If you experience "classic" migraine headaches, the kind that are preceded by an aura, you probably know it. It's hard to miss the sensory disturbances, followed by throbbing head pain. You may also know what triggers these headaches in you; they are often triggered by foods you eat, sudden changes in the weather, low blood sugar, bright or flickering lights, emotional upsets, and hormonal fluctuations. Migraine headaches, with or without aura, can last anywhere from one to seventy-two hours. The pain usually comes on gradually and can reach intense proportions. The headache generally affects one side of the head more than another, throbs or pounds, is made worse by physical movement, and may be accompanied by nausea or vomiting.

Mitral or Aortic Heart Valve Disease

Diseases or conditions that significantly affect the heart's mitral valve, the valve between the left atrium and ventricle, or the heart's aortic valve, the valve between the left ventricle and aorta, have the potential to increase ischemic stroke risk. Problems with these valves, which are on the left side of the heart and supply blood to the body, can lead to the development of clots that can travel from the heart to other areas of the body, including the brain, causing ischemic stroke. Among the conditions that can affect the mitral and aortic valves and cause clots are rheumatic heart disease, which can leave the valve deformed and damaged and cause stenosis, or narrowing; stenosis itself, which in the mitral valve increases the pressure of the blood in the left atrium and may cause the chamber to enlarge and in the aortic valve increases the pressure of blood in the left ventricle and may cause the chamber to enlarge; a replacement valve; regurgitation, in which the valve leaflets (the tiny flaps that open and close to control blood flow) do not close properly; and significant mitral valve prolapse, in which the leaflets of the valve prolapse into the left atrium when the heart contracts. Mitral valve prolapse, which is common, increases stroke risk only when it is severe.

The symptoms and diagnostic procedures for these conditions vary, and some of the conditions have no symptoms at all. For example, the vast majority of people with mitral valve prolapse do not experience symptoms, nor do many people with mitral valve stenosis. When symptoms do occur in either condition, they may include fatigue, shortness of breath, chest pain, and palpitations. Rheumatic heart disease is now rare, but since the disease was common years ago, many people have lasting damage. This damage generally manifests itself in the symptoms of mitral valve stenosis.

As for diagnosis, if you've had a valve replacement, you know it. You may also know if you had rheumatic fever as a child. Your doctor may detect other problems with the mitral or aortic valve when he or she listens to your heart through a stethoscope, or through a noninvasive test like echocardiography, which provides an image of the heart. Valve problems can also be detected with more invasive procedures like cardiac catheterization and angiography, in which a catheter is inserted into the heart and dye is injected to enhance the appearance on X rays.

Oral Contraceptives and Hormone Replacement

Controversy and conflict surround oral contraceptives and hormone replacement therapy, which involve doses of the female hormone estrogen— although for markedly different purposes.

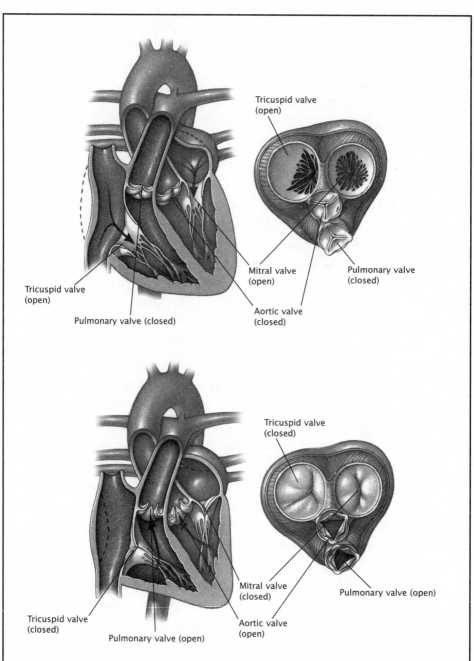

Tricuspid valve
(open)

Tricuspid valve
(open)

Pulmonary valve (closed)

Mitral valve
(open)

Aortic valve
(closed)

Pulmonary valve
(closed)

Tricuspid valve
(closed)

Tricuspid valve
(closed)

Pulmonary valve (open)

Mitral valve
(closed)

Aortic valve
(open)

Pulmonary valve (open)

Heart valves control the flow of blood, permitting it to move in only one direction. Problems with these valves, particularly the mitral and aortic valves, can lead to ischemic stroke. The mitral valve controls the flow of blood from the left atrium, or upper heart chamber, to the left ventricle, or lower chamber. The aortic valve controls the flow of blood from the left ventricle to the aorta.

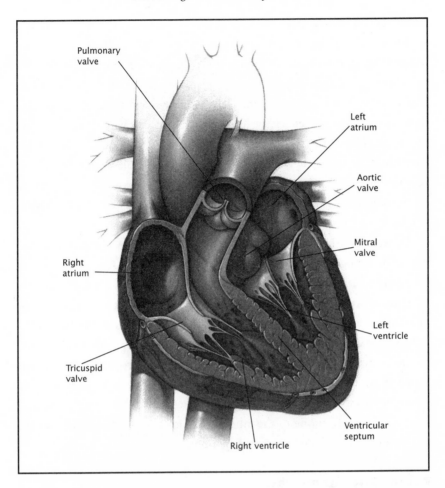

If you take oral contraceptives, you are probably aware that they have been linked to stroke. Perhaps your doctor told you, or you read on the product information label about the Pill's potential to increase the risk of blood clot formation. Most of the warnings about the Pill are based on early studies involving an older, high-estrogen version that is no longer made. The newer oral contraceptives have not been proven to be as problematic— unless a woman also smokes or has such other risk factors as hypertension. Those combinations are known to increase the risk of thromboembolism, which increases the risk of ischemic stroke, particularly the cardioembolic and "other" subtypes.

Hormone replacement, too, has been linked to increased risk of ischemic stroke. The Framingham Heart Study found that women on hormone replacement therapy were about two times more likely to have a stroke and about two and one-half times more likely to have an ischemic stroke than women who were not on the therapy. In other studies, hormone replacement therapy has been linked to a decreased risk of ischemic stroke, as well as a decreased risk of ischemic heart disease, although this link has not been proven. A Swedish study found that women on the therapy were 10 to 39 percent less likely to have a stroke than women who were not. The first U.S. National Health and Nutrition Examination Survey also found a protective effect. In that study, women on hormone replacement therapy were 31 percent less likely to have a stroke. Other studies have found no effect either way.

To me, these conflicting results can be explained by the fact that the effects of estrogen on stroke risk are related to stroke subtype. I believe estrogen increases the risk of cardioembolic stroke and the "other" subtype of ischemic stroke by increasing blood clotting. I believe it decreases the risk of ischemic stroke caused by atherosclerosis, much as it decreases the risk of ischemic heart disease. What this means is that estrogen could be problematic for women prone to cardioembolic stroke and protective for women prone to atherosclerotic stroke. The quiz takes into account only the risk conveyed by estrogen. It does not take into account the hormone's potential benefit. If you are prone to the atherosclerotic subtype of ischemic stroke, estrogen use may lower your risk of that type of stroke.

Patent Foramen Ovale

This congenital condition is an opening between the heart's right and left atria, which provides a bypass for blood that would otherwise flow into the lungs. This opening usually closes at birth, when the baby begins breathing, although it takes several months for it to close completely. In about 15 to 20 percent of people, complete closure is not achieved. This increases the likelihood that clots from the veins can make their way to the brain, causing ischemic stroke. The risk is higher depending on the severity of the opening. Some people have an opening only during straining; others have an opening at all times.

The condition is diagnosed by injecting a shaken saline solution into a vein before and after a person has performed an exercise that causes straining, then using echocardiography to watch for the appearance of bubbles in the blood as it moves from the right to left side of the heart.

Prosthetic Heart Valve

Any prosthetic or replacement heart valve, particularly those of the mitral or aortic heart valves, can increase your risk of cardioembolic ischemic stroke, particularly if you've recently experienced a TIA or minor ischemic stroke. Prosthetic heart valves replace those that have been diseased and no longer function correctly. They can significantly improve circulation and reduce the symptoms of valvular disease. At the same time, they increase the likelihood of clot development and can become infected, which can attract clots. Thus, they increase the risk of cardioembolic stroke. Prosthetic heart valves are installed during a major surgical procedure and are usually treated with long-term anticoagulant therapy. If you have a replacement heart valve, you should be treated with antibiotics before undergoing dental work and other procedures to reduce the risk of infection.

Race

Race plays only a minor role in stroke risk. Although it does not confer great risk in and of itself, it does help pinpoint the subtype of stroke for which a person is at highest risk. In general, Caucasians are more likely to experience atherosclerotic ischemic strokes and, to a lesser extent, cardioembolic and lacunar ischemic strokes, while African Americans, who have a higher likelihood of hypertension than other racial groups, are more likely to have lacunar infarctions, the type of stroke caused by hypertension. To a lesser extent, African Americans are also at risk of atherosclerotic ischemic stroke, and, because of their propensity toward sickle-cell disease, the "other" subtype of ischemic stroke. Because of their propensity to hypertension, African Americans are also at increased risk of intracerebral hemorrhage. People of Asian descent are more likely to have hemorrhagic strokes, especially subarachnoid hemorrhage. This risk appears to be related to a genetic predisposition to developing intracranial aneurysms. The background of the Hispanic community is so diverse that it has been difficult to assess across-the-board variations in risk for individuals.

The differences in stroke risk among races are probably in large part the result of genetic predisposition to or against a certain type of damage. Environmental factors may also play a role. Incidentally, this combination—genetics, environment, and race—is probably responsible for an anomaly we call the Stroke Belt. Research has found that the statistical rate of stroke is higher in an eleven-state area in the American Southeast: Alabama, Arkansas, Georgia, Indiana, Kentucky, Louisiana, Mississippi, North Carolina, South Carolina, Tennessee, and Virginia.

Recent Heart Attack

A heart attack, as you may know, is a symptom of ischemic heart disease. Like an ischemic stroke, or brain attack, it occurs when the flow of blood and oxygen—in this case, to the heart muscle, or myocardium—is obstructed, depriving an area of tissue of oxygen. If the tissue is deprived of oxygen and nutrients for a long enough time, it can die. This damage to the heart muscle—not the atherosclerosis that may be present—is the primary reason that ischemic stroke may occur within a month of a heart attack. According to autopsy studies, up to 44 percent of people who experience heart attacks develop a blood clot in their left ventricle as a result of the damage. In some cases, these clots make their way to the brain, causing cardioembolic stroke.

Depending on the size and severity of a heart attack, you may or may not know you've had one. Some people experience few or only passing symptoms, such as a transitory chest pain that they may mistake for angina. Others feel the traditional crushing pain in the chest that we've all heard about. Symptoms of heart attack include pain, or pressure, in the chest that may radiate to the left arm, pain in the upper abdomen, shortness of breath, pale skin, sweating, vomiting, and loss of consciousness. These symptoms—like the symptoms of brain attack—are your cue to get to the emergency room as soon as possible. There, your doctor may diagnose your heart attack based on your symptoms, history, and a number of tests, including blood tests for cardiac enzymes that may indicate damage from a heart attack; electrocardiography (ECG or EKG), which can show your heart rhythm and indicate that a part of the heart has been damaged; echocardiography, which can show damage to the heart muscle; and nuclear scans, which can provide information about your heart's pumping ability and blood flow to the heart muscle.

Rheumatic Heart Disease

Rheumatic heart disease is the result of rheumatic fever, a serious infection that was once common in the United States. The disease, caused by infection with certain strains of the Streptococcus bacteria, often appeared in the wake of an untreated bout of "strep throat," a common throat infection marked by sore throat, fever, and swollen glands. Widespread treatment of strep throat with antibiotics in recent decades has made rheumatic fever much less common. However, it still appears from time to time, and many people who had the disease when they were younger still experience problems as a result.

You may have had rheumatic fever in your youth if you experienced fever, chills, joint pains, rash, a rapid heartbeat, fatigue, weakness, and irritability in the weeks after what seemed to be a typical throat infection. Since having the fever makes you more susceptible to another attack, you may have taken antibiotics until adulthood to prevent a recurrence. The primary problem with rheumatic fever, as it relates to the heart, is its propensity to inflame the heart valves. This inflammation can lead to scarring and permanent damage that may take years to become obvious but may ultimately result in valvular heart disease and valve replacement surgery.

Sick Sinus Syndrome

Sick sinus syndrome has nothing to do with breathing or headaches; it's a collection of symptoms caused by problems in the heart's sinus node, or natural pacemaker. The sinus, or sinoatrial, node generates the heartbeat by sending an electrical impulse through the left atrium. In this capacity, it is responsible for maintaining a normal heart rhythm. Sometimes, however, the sinus node fails to function properly. It may pause too long between beats, initiate beats more slowly, or stop producing beats. These malfunctions of the sinus node are referred to as sick sinus syndrome. Sick sinus syndrome may result in a slow, fast, or irregular heartbeat and symptoms including fatigue, shortness of breath, light-headedness, and palpitations (racing or pounding heartbeat). Any of these symptoms may lead your doctor to test for heart rhythm abnormalities, including sick sinus syndrome. The condition may also show up on a routine electrocardiogram.

Sickle-Cell Disease

Sickle-cell disease is an inherited disease that primarily affects African Americans and other people of African descent. It can also affect Hispanics from the Caribbean and non-Hispanics from the Mediterranean region and Middle East. In sickle-cell disease, the red blood cells develop a curved, or sickle, shape. They can break up, leading to the development of anemia, and they can block vessels and impair circulation, causing pain and, if they impair circulation to the brain, ischemic stroke. Not all people with sickle-cell disease will experience ischemic strokes. Ischemic stroke is an infrequent complication of sickle-cell disease; nevertheless, the disease is a leading cause of ischemic stroke in children. The average age at which a child with sickle-cell disease has a stroke is seven.

To develop sickle-cell disease, you must inherit a defective gene called sickle-cell trait from both your parents. The trait itself rarely results in symptoms. Symptoms of sickle-cell disease include rapid heart rate, enlarged heart and liver, heart murmurs, fatigue, shortness of breath, jaundice (a yellowing of the skin), joint swelling, and painful episodes called sickle-cell crises. Your doctor will diagnose the condition based on your symptoms and your family history. If both of your parents have the disease, you will have it. If both of your parents are simply carriers, you have a 25 percent chance of having the disease. A blood test can determine whether or not you have this genetic defect.

Smoking

That smoking is a risk factor for stroke should come as no surprise. No doubt you know that smoking is associated with ischemic heart disease and atherosclerosis. It also affects the blood, making it thicker and more likely to clot, and it raises blood pressure. As a result, it increases the risk of all types of ischemic stroke. Smoking presents an increased risk in women who use oral contraceptives or hormone replacement therapy. The combination can predispose a woman to develop blood clots that can make their way into the blood vessels of the brain and cause ischemic stroke.

In addition, we have recently determined that smoking contributes to the development of intracranial aneurysms. In fact, multiple intracranial aneurysms become more likely. Although we haven't established whether smoking causes these outpouchings to rupture, the fact that it contributes to their development makes it a risk factor for both subarachnoid and intracerebral hemorrhage.

Secondhand smoke, too, increases the risk of all types of stroke. Fortunately, smoking cessation or avoiding secondhand smoke decreases risk rapidly. Five years after quitting, a smoker's risk is similar to that of a person who never smoked.

Stress and/or Stimulant Drugs

Hormones released during stress have been found to increase heart rate and blood pressure. Studies indicate that one of these hormones, cortisol, raises blood cholesterol levels and accelerates the development of atherosclerosis. Few studies have focused on stress as a risk factor for stroke, but it has been implicated as a risk factor in ischemic heart disease. The cardiovascular changes stress hormones produce can affect stroke risk.

Stress and other psychological factors, including excessive anxiety, hostility, and anger, can also contribute to hypertension, which increases the risk of both lacunar ischemic stroke and intracerebral hemorrhage. Surprisingly, hypertension is not a risk factor for subarachnoid hemorrhage.

Short-term, temporary, rapid increases in blood pressure are another story. Blood pressure fluctuates regularly. In most cases, a transitory jump is nothing to worry about. If you have an aneurysm or vascular malformation, there is some evidence that a rapid spike in blood pressure may cause it to rupture. These rapid, temporary spikes in blood pressure may be caused by any of a number of factors, including stress or anxiety, physical activity, and various substances with stimulant effects. Examples include certain prescription medications, such street drugs as cocaine and amphetamines, some decongestants and cold medicines (phenylpropanolamine preparations were taken off the market in late 2000 because of concerns about increased risk of hemorrhagic stroke), and, to a lesser extent, even our most widely used "upper," caffeine. The evidence isn't strong enough for me to ask you to give up your morning coffee, but you might want to switch to decaf if you're at risk of hemorrhagic stroke.

Transient Ischemic Attack/Minor Ischemic Stroke

Transient ischemic attack, or TIA, is perhaps the most telltale sign of ischemic stroke risk. A TIA is essentially a mini-stroke—an emergency event in its own right. If you have had a TIA, you are clearly at risk for a full-blown event—of any ischemic stroke subtype. Across the board, between 30 and 40 percent of people who experience these strokelike events ultimately have an ischemic stroke. The risk may be even higher among people with other risk factors. The actual risk related to these events depends on how recently and how many times they occurred.

In a TIA, the blood supply to an area of the brain is temporarily interrupted, causing strokelike symptoms that last less than twenty-four hours. These symptoms may include:

- sudden numbness or weakness in the face, arm, or leg, particularly on one side of the body
- sudden blurred or decreased vision or sudden double vision
- sudden difficulty speaking or understanding others
- sudden dizziness, loss of balance, or loss of coordination.

These symptoms can be minor or severe.

Since the only distinctions between TIA and ischemic stroke are the duration of symptoms and the reversible nature, a TIA requires immediate diagnosis and treatment. Until you know how long your symptoms last, you will not know whether you've had a TIA; a similar event called a reversible ischemic neurologic deficit (RIND), in which symptoms resolve between twenty-four hours and three weeks; a minor cerebral infarction; or a minor ischemic stroke, in which the symptoms are permanent, but minor; or a major ischemic stroke.

All of these events are diagnosed in the same manner as stroke. The doctor will ask about your personal and family medical history as well as your symptoms: what they include, when they started, how quickly they came on, when they resolved (if they did), and so on. The doctor will also conduct a physical examination that includes a neurologic component. He or she will observe your behavior and movement, test your reflexes, listen to you speak, test your mental function, and perform a variety of other tests to determine what area of the brain may be affected and to what extent. The doctor will also take your blood pressure, listen to your heart, check your breathing, and perform other standard examination procedures. Depending on the results of this exam and whether or not the symptoms persist, the doctor may recommend an imaging test like computed tomography or magnetic resonance imaging to see what's going on in your brain. Blood tests may also be performed.

Ultimately, time and the severity of any lasting symptoms play a role in the diagnosis. If the symptoms resolve within a few hours, you've had a TIA; if the symptoms persist but resolve within three weeks, you've had a RIND; if the symptoms never resolve, but are minor, you've had a minor cerebral infarction; and if the symptoms persist and are severe, you've had a major ischemic stroke. Even when these events are minor, they greatly increase your risk of having a major ischemic stroke. Your risk is highest in the first four weeks after the TIA or other event, especially if you've had more than one event in that time period.

Although the risk conveyed by a TIA or minor ischemic stroke decreases with time, it remains high within the first year after the event. The risk is extremely high within the first few months of the event if the event occurred in conjunction with another known risk factor. Among these risk factors are a high-grade stenosis, or narrowing, of the carotid artery, which increases the risk of atherosclerotic ischemic stroke; heart conditions such as atrial fibrillation, congestive heart failure, prosthetic heart valves, recent heart attack, sick sinus syndrome, mitral valve disease, a clot in the heart, a ventricular aneurysm, or a recent heart attack, which increase the risk of cardioembolic stroke; and chronic hypertension, particularly above 200/110 mm Hg, which increases the risk of lacunar stroke.

If you think you may have had a TIA, RIND, or minor ischemic stroke but did not report to the doctor or hospital when the event occurred, talk about your experience with your doctor or a doctor with expertise in cerebrovascular disorders. These events are among the strongest risk factors for ischemic stroke and greatly affect your overall risk.

Vascular Malformations

A vascular malformation is exactly what the term implies: a malformation of blood vessels. When these congenital malformations of blood vessels occur in the brain, they have potential to rupture, causing intracerebral hemorrhage, or less commonly, subarachnoid hemorrhage. Several types of vascular malformations exist. The type that most commonly causes hemorrhagic stroke is the arteriovenous malformation, or AVM, a grouping of thin-walled blood vessels that includes arteries, veins, and other blood vessels that appear to be a cross between arteries and veins. Other problem malformations include cavernous malformations, benign, blood-filled tumors; venous malformations, or malformations of veins; and dural-based arteriovenous fistulae, arteries that cover the layer of the brain known as the dura.

Like intracranial aneurysms, vascular malformations generally exhibit no symptoms and generally remain undetected unless they rupture or unless they are detected during an imaging test conducted for another purpose or condition. On rare occasions, these malformations can produce a warning leak similar to those produced by unruptured intracranial aneurysms. These leaks are characterized by seizures, sudden, severe headache that may resemble a migraine, a stiff neck, nausea, vomiting, and an aversion to light. Vascular malformations can also cause symptoms as they grow and impinge on brain tissue. These symptoms pose less of an immediate threat than those caused by a warning leak but should be checked out nonetheless. They include seizures, migrainelike symptoms, and temporary or progressive neurological problems such as numbness or weakness on one side and tinnitus (ringing in the ears).

Ventricular Aneurysm

A (heart) ventricular aneurysm, like an intracranial aneurysm, is an outpouching, or ballooning. In this case, it's a ballooning of a section of muscle in one of the ventricles, or lower chambers, of the heart. Ventricular aneurysms are generally complications of a heart attack. They can affect the heart's ability to pump blood and trigger rhythm disorders. They can also trigger the formation of blood clots. Again, because ventricular aneurysms often require treatment and generally follow a serious condition like heart attack, you'll likely know if you've been diagnosed with one.

4

Preventing Your Stroke

I've spent the better part of my career reacting to stroke. In fact, stroke has introduced me to many of my patients. I met them as they arrived at the hospital suffering from stroke symptoms, or a short time later, and did what I could to help them recover. I've had many successes. I've seen patients survive to overcome the initial deficits caused by stroke or to adjust to the deficits that remain.

Unfortunately, I've also had failures. I've seen some patients die, and others be robbed of life as they knew it. Regardless of the outcome, I've wished I could have met these people before they had strokes. Perhaps if I had, I could have done something to prevent the event. Perhaps together we could have faced stroke before it attacked, rather than after. I guess every physician dreams of preventing the diseases he or she treats.

THE PARADOX OF PREVENTION: OVERCOMING PSYCHOLOGICAL BARRIERS TO CHANGE

Until now, that dream has remained elusive for those of us who treat stroke. To be sure, we've made progress. As we've gained insight into the various causes of stroke, we've also learned how to prevent it. Though our medical sophistication about stroke prevention has grown, our ability to prevent stroke hasn't kept pace. I've written this book to speed the dissemination of prevention information—and motivation—that people need to overcome their natural tendency to avoid warning signs until it's too late.

85

Our initial prevention efforts centered around treating underlying conditions that could lead to stroke and in following a "heart-healthy" lifestyle to reduce the risk of heart disease and to maintain the health of the vascular system, which is, of course, tied to the brain as well as the heart. This was a logical and useful place to start. The public's interest in heart disease prevention has focused attention on the dangers of smoking, the need to control blood pressure, and the importance of a low-fat, low-cholesterol diet. We simply had to spread the word that these lifestyle choices—and others—are also important for brain health, although for different reasons.

Some people have gotten the message, but most have not. A 1996 survey conducted by the Gallup Organization for the National Stroke Association found that 38 percent of Americans age fifty or older do not know where in the body a stroke occurs, and only 19 percent of Americans are aware that there are things they can do to help prevent stroke.

Although the medical community and the government could certainly be doing more to promote prevention education, I think the problem runs deeper than that. It's fundamentally a mind-over-matter problem. Much has been written about mind/body medicine, but I feel that if we are sincere about prevention, we first need to confront the ways our minds—emotionally and psychologically—can work against our best health interests.

On a purely physical level, preventive medicine is no different from preventive maintenance of our cars, houses, or appliances. We all know intellectually that if we don't change the oil in our car or change the furnace filter every season or so, we'll soon be facing much more expensive, and potentially dangerous, repairs. In fact, most of us take better care of our cars and houses than we do of our bodies, these infinitely precious and irreplaceable vessels that sustain our consciousness. Most adults now understand that smoking and heavy drinking and a high-fat diet are likely to shorten their lives significantly. Yet we are seeing obesity rates soar as fatty fast food continues to dominate our food culture, alcohol's popularity never seems to wane, and tens of millions of us still smoke.

What's going on here? In a word: denial.

Biologists and psychologists concur that we are creatures of pleasure. We're wired that way, from infancy onward. It's very difficult to acknowledge that the activities we've come to depend on for pleasure are bad for us—even in the face of irrefutable scientific evidence. Children don't want to hear that sugar is bad for their teeth. Adults are often equally resistant to the health consequences of some of their favorite foods and drinks.

On a deeper level, we are in denial of our own mortality. At one time in our distant past, this may well have been an evolutionary advantage—we couldn't get much accomplished if we stood around all day worrying about being eaten by wild animals. When we were living on the African savanna millennia ago, there were scarce supplies of fat, no tobacco, not much in the way of fermented beverages. Today, cheeseburgers and french fries are low-hanging fruit available at every street corner, as are beer and cigarettes. We are not biologically engineered to live on high-meat, high-fat, fast-food diets—or to smoke or drink a lot—and our vascular systems are paying the price.

Ultimately, it is and needs to be each patient's choice on these issues. Life without pleasure would be a whole lot less fun. But it pains me deeply to watch people forfeit decades of health and function to what in many cases amount to addictions. I'll never forget a vibrant woman in her early fifties who came to our clinic with a subarachnoid hemorrhage. Susan was a talented singer who had been enjoying a revival in her career after a decade-long lull—when an aneurysm ruptured in her head. She was in a coma when she initially arrived at the hospital, and only about 20 percent of people who arrive in that condition survive, much less recover. Susan was one of the lucky ones. We ultimately found the aneurysm, and we were able to repair it surgically. She made a strong recovery. After three months of rehabilitation, she began working again.

Before she left the hospital, she and I reviewed the lifestyle changes she'd have to make to stay healthy. Cigarettes were at the top of her list of risk factors for aneurysms and hemorrhagic stroke. She'd been at two packs a day ever since her early twenties. Susan had woven cigarettes into the fabric of her life, particularly her work routine. Despite spending time in a smoking cessation program with follow-up support back home, Susan wasn't able to kick her habit. Five years later, following a performance in a successful musical, Susan had another ruptured aneurysm. She died before the ambulance reached the hospital.

For every tragedy like Susan's, I can point to numerous stories of patients who have taken control of their lives and turned a bad prognosis into long life. I've made a point of studying what seems to motivate people to overcome our natural human desire to deny and ignore warning signs of stroke.

For some, the scare of a near-death experience makes them reorder their priorities. I remember a high-powered chief executive named Jack who came to me after a series of TIAs. He had the classic high-stress profile: hypertension, bad diet, chest pains, plus a bad family history. When I told him that his high-stress lifestyle was killing him, he sat in silence for a full minute, then broke down in tears. All his life he had worked hard for the recognition and status his job afforded him, but it wasn't having to change his work habits that moved him to tears. Opening his wallet, Jack proudly displayed a photo of his daughter's newborn baby boy, his first grandchild. Jack confided to me, "I worked like a demon when my own kids were young. I hardly knew them. I've been planning on making it up to them by being the world's best grandfather." Now he was terrified of never seeing his first grandchild grow up.

Resolved to turn his life around, Jack's dogged determination became his best ally for a change. Together we worked out a regimen of medications, exercise, and diet, and he stuck to it religiously. He also cut out most of his work-related travel and stopped working weekends. His risk factors gradually abated, and his quality of life improved. The last time I saw him, Jack was showing off a picture of himself with his twelve-year-old grandson on a camping trip.

For many people, embracing prevention means finding a metaphor that has meaning on a personal level. I had a patient who was a civil engineer for the highway department. After spending about forty-five minutes listening to me explain that his family history of hardened arteries had put him at risk for ischemic stroke, a light went on in his head. "I get it. It's just like road maintenance. If you wait till you get potholes, you'll be patching and filling till the cows come home. But if you're repaving regularly every seven years, you'll always have good roads." I've had plumbers who have latched on to plumbing metaphors, a car mechanic who saw his cerebrovascular system reflected in a car's fuel lines, and an architect who understood her risk of hemorrhagic stroke as an overpressurized heating and air conditioning system. Other patients, like Jack, are more effectively motivated by a fear of loss of loved ones or a sense of responsibility to people who depend on them, whether husbands, children, or coworkers.

The point is to find the psychological wedge that works best for you, because prevention doesn't come naturally. You have to identify the rewards and work toward them. It's tough to accept that our bodies are fragile and fleeting organisms. In these days of genome supremacy, it's easy to get trapped in genetic fatalism: "If I've got bad genes, there's nothing I can do about it." But genes are not a life or death sentence. They are only part of the picture—a forecast of what could happen if you don't take preventive steps. I've had many, many patients who recognized a bad family history as a risk factor they had to deal with and used that realization to extend and improve their lives. We each have a large measure of control over our health and longevity—if we can translate what we know into action.

There's so much to be excited about in stroke prevention today. We have a much greater understanding of cerebrovascular disease and an impressive arsenal of preventive treatments. There are new surgical techniques, amazing new medications, and groundbreaking research about how lifestyle changes can arrest—and in the case of some risk factors like atherosclerosis, actually reverse—the course of cerebrovascular disease.

So let's get started preventing your stroke!

TAKING THE NEXT STEP

By completing the risk assessment test, you've already taken the first step toward prevention. Now that you've tallied the results, you probably have a lot of questions and emotions running through your mind. This can be a scary time, especially if you've found you are at moderate or high risk of having a stroke. You're now ready for the second step: educating yourself about what you can do to reduce your risk and working with your doctor to design your personal prescription for stroke prevention.

If your score on the assessment shows that you are at low risk for stroke, you can skip this chapter altogether and go straight to chapter 5: "The Stroke-Free for Life Prevention Plan." That chapter will offer you lifestyle guidelines for keeping your risk low, even as you age. You can implement that plan without any medical supervision, unless you're on medication, in which case you should consult with your doctor.

If you are at moderate to high risk, use this chapter to educate yourself about the preventive treatment options for each individual risk factor—from such high-tech interventions as gamma knife radiosurgery to simple lifestyle modifications. I'll be reviewing benefits and possible risks of each option, and, whenever possible, give you my opinion about which treatments are preferable and why. Remember, my goal isn't to make decisions for you, and it's certainly not to replace the role of your own doctor. My goal is to provide you with the information you need to walk into your doctor's office as a fully informed partner. Together you can address your specific risk factors and work out a personalized prevention program.

The treatment options for risk factors are discussed in alphabetical order under the same risk factor headings as in chapter 3. (You only need to read the sections that are relevant to your risk factors.) I explain what treatments are available for each risk factor, starting with surgical interventions, then moving to medications, then to lifestyle modifications. This progression isn't meant to imply that the high-tech treatments are the most effective; it's simply a logical way to organize the information. As I've said earlier, the simplest solution can sometimes be the best. It is usually preferable to start with the least invasive, most natural approach and work your way into higher-tech treatments if you need them, except in certain situations, such as if your underlying condition is severe or your immediate stroke risk is extremely high. In fact, I strongly favor a noninvasive approach whenever possible, especially when the high-tech diagnostic or therapeutic approach is associated with risk. (The most memorable phrase for me in the Hippocratic Oath is: "First, do no harm.") Lifestyle modifications reduce the likelihood of complications and side effects and enhance the body's natural healing abilities. There are times when more invasive measures are necessary, and in those cases, I'm always grateful that we have so many good surgical and drug treatments from which to choose.

The most important guiding principle in developing a prevention plan should be pragmatism. Whatever works, is safe, and fits best with your personal preferences should be considered. Being rigidly for or against any given treatment modality (whether surgery, medications, or lifestyle modifications) is counterproductive. An ideal regimen will weigh each treatment option on its merits and find the best combination for you.

After you've read about the treatment options for your risk factors in this chapter, I suggest you also read about the stroke-free lifestyle plan in chapter 5, which will serve as a preventive maintenance program once you've treated your moderate-to-high risk factors. Then schedule an appointment with your doctor. Take along your completed assessment and this book, and let them serve as a guide in your discussion about how to address your risk factors. Good doctors want their patients to be educated about their conditions, and since few of them have the time to brief you on all the details, they'll appreciate all the research you've done. After all, much of the work of implementing your plan—and all of the final decision-making—is up to you. Patients are more likely to follow a prescribed regimen if they've had some say in designing it around their own personal likes, dislikes, fears, and feelings.

Your input—as well as your own personal history and risk—should play a crucial role in creating your personal stroke prevention prescription. Given what we now know about stroke, stroke prevention, by its very nature, should be individual. Each person has his or her own unique set of risk factors, factors that make him or her more vulnerable to particular types of stroke. And each risk factor can be addressed in a number of ways. A standard, one-size-fits-all prescription is no longer acceptable.

Here is the order and page number of the risk factors discussed in this chapter:

THE PREVENTION TOOLBOX: A BRIEF OVERVIEW

I'll be discussing the various treatment modalities under the specific risk factor headings later in this chapter. For now, let me just give you a brief overview of the types of tools that you and your doctor have at your disposal.

Stroke prevention is on the verge of revolution not only because we can now tailor our efforts to individuals, but also because we have more preventive tools than ever at our disposal. Stroke prevention tools, like those you find at a hardware store, come in many forms. There are high-tech commercial tools (for which you generally have to call in an expert) like surgery, potent power tools like medication, and simple-but-effective hand tools, like lifestyle changes. A self-improvement project like stroke prevention may require a combination of tools from various categories. As with a home improvement project, not all tools may be appropriate. You don't need a commercial band saw to cut a small dowel, for instance. And sometimes a fine hand sanding results in a better finish than a power sanding. Still, it's nice to know that the high-tech tools are available when you need them. The same holds true in stroke prevention. The high-tech procedures the medical community has developed—and continues to develop—bring new energy and excitement to our prevention efforts. For many people, simple lifestyle changes like smoking cessation can have an even greater effect. Fortunately, we can choose from—and combine—tools of every technology level to achieve our goal.

Surgical/Interventional: The High-Tech Tools

At the top of the technology level are surgery and interventional procedures designed to address the underlying risk factors and causes of ischemic and hemorrhagic stroke. Needless to say, their applicability to a stroke prevention program depends on the type of stroke for which a person is at risk and that person's individual risk factors. These tools range from brain surgery, heart surgery, and high-tech radiation therapies like gamma knife radiosurgery to cardioversion shock treatments and pacemakers. They are strong medicine and must be used with caution.

Medications: The Power Tools

Medications may not be as dramatic as surgical procedures, but they can be extremely effective stroke prevention tools. In fact, they're as essential to the stroke prevention toolbox as the electric drill, power sander, and circular saw are to the home improvement expert's. These power tools have been staples of heart, hypertension, and diabetes treatment for years. New formulations and uses come out regularly, constantly expanding our treatment options. As we uncover links between stroke and other conditions, these options are proliferating rapidly.

The choice of drug to treat a particular condition—and to prevent stroke—should be tailored to the individual. I discuss the factors that go into choosing an appropriate medication later in the chapter, but you need to work with your doctor to find the most appropriate medication.

Lifestyle Changes: Tried and True Hand Tools

The least high-tech of the stroke prevention tools are lifestyle changes, but don't let their low-tech nature fool you. These tools are often the most powerful and most healthy of all. The way you live your life can dictate your stroke risk. If you smoke and eat a high-fat diet, for example, you not only have two immediate risk factors for stroke, you're also well on your way to others, including atherosclerosis, hypertension, heart disease, and unruptured aneurysm. Although stroke appears to come out of the blue, more times than not, it is the result of a lifetime of bad habits. Fortunately, reversing those habits—or making a conscious effort to follow a healthy lifestyle—can have a profound impact on stroke risk.

BEYOND ONE-SIZE-FITS-ALL

Not too long ago, the best advice we could offer people was a one-size-fits-all prescription for stroke prevention: avoid smoking, control blood pressure, eat a healthy diet, and follow the recommended treatment for any potentially stroke-causing conditions they have. We might also have advised them to take an aspirin a day. On the surface, there's really nothing wrong with this advice. For many people, it's valid. For some, it can be—and has been—lifesaving.

But it doesn't go far enough, and, for some people, it is downright misleading. Take, for example, a middle-aged woman who has a family history of intracranial aneurysms. She doesn't smoke, doesn't have high blood pressure or any other known condition, and eats a relatively healthy diet. That leaves her with one option from the one-size-fits-all prescription: taking a daily aspirin. Aspirin offers some protection against ischemic stroke, particularly for people with atherosclerosis, but it does nothing to prevent hemorrhagic stroke. In fact, it could make it difficult to stop bleeding after a rupture has occurred and, at least in theory, could even promote a hemorrhage. Her family history indicates that she is at some risk for having an aneurysm. She may be more likely to have a hemorrhagic stroke than an ischemic stroke, which means the aspirin regimen may do her more harm than good.

The one-size-fits-all prescription for stroke prevention, like much of the research into risk factors, doesn't take stroke subtype into account, nor does it take into account other factors unique to an individual. Let's look at Harold. He's seventy-five and has hypertension, which puts him at increased risk of ischemic stroke and of intracerebral hemorrhage. We cannot change his age and gender, so we have to focus on controlling his hypertension with medication. The number of available antihypertensive medications is staggering and continues to grow. Choosing the right one is important. Some of the medications available are harmful in the presence of other problems; others offer additional protection. Medications known as ACE inhibitors, for example, may help prevent ischemic stroke independent of their role in reducing blood pressure, but these drugs are not appropriate for people with certain kidney problems.

Obviously, we have to look at a number of factors before we simply prescribe an ACE inhibitor for Harold. Does he have a personal or family history of kidney problems? Is he at greater risk of ischemic stroke or of hemorrhagic stroke? Does he have any heart conditions that could benefit from the medication? The answers to these questions are crucial to determining which treatment is most appropriate for him. Another man the same age with the same level of hypertension may benefit more from a different medication.

As you can see, stroke prevention needs to be tailored to the individual. It should also take into account a person's preferences and viewpoints. After all, no matter what your individual stroke prevention program entails, you have a major role in its success or failure. Your doctor can order procedures, prescribe medications, and advise you of lifestyle changes that can reduce your risk of stroke, but it's up to you to follow through—to agree to a procedure, to take your medication, to change your diet. To be successful, a stroke prevention program must be a partnership between doctor and patient.

David is a good example. When the fifty-seven-year-old legal aid attorney came to see me, he had hypertension, ischemic heart disease, occasional chest pain, and TIA-like spells. This hardworking man became emotionally involved with many of his clients, which was the main reason he was so stressed out by his day-to-day work. Together, we developed a morning physical exercise program for him, and a program of relaxation exercises for his afternoon lunch break. I also advised him to reduce his daily caffeine intake from ten cups per day to two or less. It was up to him to follow through. And it was his decision alone to take other initiatives to reduce his stress level, cutting his caseload, for example. Our combined efforts paid off. He lowered his blood pressure, eliminated his chest pains, and has not had a TIA in five years.

A Word of Explanation About Stroke Subtypes

As you can see from the above examples, knowing the subtype or subtypes of stroke to which you are susceptible is critical information for creating an individual approach to prevention. One reason the assessment questionnaire in this book is particularly helpful—and different from previous prevention profilers—is because it gives you an overall risk score for stroke and a risk score by stroke subtype.

Although you should address all of your modifiable risk factors, you should pay special attention to those factors that increase the risk of your particular subtype. I'll give you the specific guidance you need later in this chapter. For example, if you know you are particularly prone to cardioembolic ischemic stroke, you should consider avoiding hormone replacement therapy or oral contraceptives, because they could add to your cardioembolic stroke risk. On the other hand, if you are prone to atherosclerotic ischemic stroke, you might want to consider taking these same medications, because they could reduce your atherosclerotic stroke risk.

BEYOND RISK REDUCTION

Stroke prevention through risk reduction is a reality. We've now set our sights on a new goal: risk factor prevention. Imagine being able to prevent the development of risk factors! It's not a far-fetched dream.

To some extent, we already promote this idea. We tell people to eat a healthy diet and to exercise regularly to stay healthy. We simply need to be more specific. For example, we know that a low-fat, low-cholesterol diet helps prevent the buildup of atherosclerotic plaque in the arteries, a major cause of ischemic stroke. Therefore, we need to tell people that following a low-fat diet throughout life can help *prevent* the development of such ischemic stroke risk factors as atherosclerosis, high cholesterol, and ischemic heart disease. Likewise, we've recently discovered that smoking contributes to the development of intracranial aneurysms, a risk factor for hemorrhagic stroke. We need to pass the word that smoking cessation or, better yet, never smoking, can help *prevent* the development of intracranial aneurysms.

Research is doing wonders to take this approach even further. A growing body of evidence indicates that problems in the endothelium, the layer of cells that line the insides of blood vessels, play a role in the development of atherosclerosis. Our research team of cardiologists and neurologists at Mayo Clinic has identified a way to predict when an individual has a high risk of developing various risk factors, including atrial fibrillation and congestive heart failure, leading causes of cardioembolic stroke. This insight will help in stroke prevention. It will help us identify people who may be at increased risk of various types of stroke so that we can tailor a prevention program to their individual risk factors, both existing and predicted. This could be our biggest advance ever in prevention. It has the potential to affect a huge number of people.

In time, these high-risk individuals may even be able to take medication to prevent these risk factors from developing. This would revolutionize stroke prevention and could help make the third leading cause of death an uncommon occurrence.

Some of these risk prevention approaches are incorporated into this chapter. The more speculative approaches that still lie in the future are covered in chapter 8, which looks at stroke prevention breakthroughs on the near horizon.

Alcohol

Although light to moderate drinking may decrease the risk of atherosclerotic ischemic stroke, heavy alcohol use and binge drinking are associated with hemorrhagic stroke and cardioembolic ischemic stroke. If you drink heavily or you are inclined to go on binges of heavy drinking, you should consider cutting back, abstaining, or changing your drinking behavior to reduce your risk of stroke, particularly if you are at risk of hemorrhagic or cardioembolic ischemic stroke. Unfortunately, this is not always easy to do. Alcohol is a drug, a drug on which people can become physically and emotionally dependent. For some people, cutting back on drinking or quitting altogether is simply a matter of deciding to do so and following through. For others, the solution requires outside help—from medical professionals, a support group, or both.

Alcohol consumption is clearly a lifestyle factor, but treatments for alcohol abuse include medical treatments as well as lifestyle changes. This is because alcoholism is a disease. Alcohol can produce a physical dependency that can trigger physical symptoms and mental symptoms like depression when the drug is withdrawn. Treatment for alcoholism and alcohol abuse can take place in a residential treatment program, in an outpatient treatment program, or through counseling sessions and support groups.

MEDICAL

If you are physically dependent upon alcohol, your treatment may begin in a detoxification unit and may include medications to help you move through the withdrawal process. Alcohol withdrawal can produce depression, agitation, a mild increase in pulse, blood pressure, and body temperature, nausea, diarrhea, and other gastrointestinal discomfort. It can also cause a mild case of the "shakes." These symptoms generally last about three to five days. Some people may have additional problems, including nightmares, anxiety, panic attacks, confusion, hallucinations, trembling, paranoia, and even seizures. These symptoms, known as delirium tremens, or the DTs, also last about three to five days, although they can sometimes last longer. Short-term medical treatment with tranquilizers, usually benzodiazepines like Valium, and, in some cases, antidepressants can help prevent these symptoms or help you deal with them. These medications are discussed in more detail in the "Depression" and "Stress" sections in this chapter.

Medication is also available to help people who have quit drinking remain sober. Two medications, disulfiram (Antabuse) and naltrexone (ReVia), are available. Antabuse discourages drinking by causing nausea, vomiting, and other unpleasant symptoms whenever alcohol is used. ReVia helps lessen the craving for alcohol.

LIFESTYLE

Lifestyle plays a major role in treating alcoholism—from becoming motivated enough to cut back on drinking, to determining when and why you drink, to seeking counseling.

Motivation

Cutting back on alcohol requires motivation. One of the best ways to start is to list your reasons for cutting down or stopping. Your overall health is one reason. Heavy alcohol use has numerous negative effects on the body in addition to increasing stroke risk. You may also have personal and social reasons to quit drinking. If you're not sure whether you have a problem, keep a diary of the number and types of drinks you consume each day. Your family members and friends may be able to provide you with additional reasons. As you cut back, your improved health and well-being may provide you with additional motivation.

Acceptance

Another prerequisite for conquering alcohol abuse—one that can give you motivation—is accepting that you have a problem. Alcoholism is a disease, an addiction to alcohol. It is not a lack of willpower or strength. You need to accept the fact that you are suffering from a powerful disease in order to seek—and succeed in—treatment. This is the first and most important step in recovery.

Cutting Back

Although some people require help—including medical treatment—to cut back on or quit drinking alcohol, others are able to cut back by adopting one or more of the following strategies.

- Set a limit—or goal—for how much you want to drink. Write down the goal, and keep track of your drinking using a diary.
- Cut back gradually. Try to avoid drinking at all one or two days each week. Next, try to stop for a week.
- Don't keep alcohol at home.
- Just say no. You don't have to drink when everyone else is drinking.
- Be aware of when you drink and why, and try to avoid temptation. If

you always drink when you're out with a certain group of friends, avoid them or devise a plan to keep you from drinking when you are with them. If you drink when you're hungry, eat something. Find other satisfying hobbies and social activities.

• When you drink, sip slowly. Don't drink to quench your thirst. Do not drink on an empty stomach. And follow an alcoholic beverage with a nonalcoholic beverage.

Counseling

Alcohol abuse affects your social and emotional health as well as your physical health. In many cases, people turn to alcohol in response to another problem—physical or emotional. Counseling—either individual or group—can help you cope with the underlying problems that trigger your drinking as well as the problems your drinking causes. It can also help you cope with abstention and restore relationships that may have been damaged when you were abusing alcohol.

Continuing Support

Your success after recovery depends in large part on the support you receive. Your family can help you here, as can a support and self-help group such as Alcoholics Anonymous. Most experts believe alcoholism cannot yet be cured. This means that even if you have been sober for a long time, you may have a relapse. For this reason, you need to both avoid alcohol and seek continuing support.

Anticoagulants/Other Blood-Thinning Drugs

The use of anticoagulants and other blood-thinning drugs increases the risk of hemorrhagic stroke. This should come as no surprise: the drugs are designed to facilitate blood flow, and hemorrhage essentially amounts to blood flow outside the blood vessels. These medications, which include anticoagulants like heparin and warfarin (Coumadin, Panwarfin) and thrombolytic, or clot-busting, medications like tissue plasminogen activator (tPA), streptokinase, and urokinase, can be lifesavers if you have ischemic heart disease or ischemic stroke. However, they can cause hemorrhage in the brain. In many cases, this potential risk pales in comparison to failure to treat the condition for which the medication is prescribed. In some instances, it may be possible to use another medication to treat the condition. For example, in some cases, your doctor may be able to substitute an antiplatelet agent like aspirin or clopidogrel, which thins the blood but in a less profound way and does not convey the same amount of bleeding risk. Check with your doctor to see if a substitution is possible, particularly if you have any other risk factors for hemorrhagic stroke.

In addition, be aware that vitamin K counteracts the effects of warfarin and makes it difficult to control the thinness of the blood. If you are taking warfarin, avoid taking in excessive amounts of vitamin K, which is found in dark greens including kale, spinach, turnip greens, lettuce, watercress, and parsley, as well as broccoli, brussels sprouts, carrots, cucumbers, avocados, leeks, and olive, canola, and soybean oils. You should also avoid multivitamin supplements that contain vitamin K. See the box below for more advice.

Ironically, if an anticoagulant medication makes your blood too thin, vitamin K can be given to reverse its effects quickly. Another treatment for thin blood is fresh frozen plasma.

Factors That Affect Oral Anticoagulant Therapy

Oral anticoagulant therapy, warfarin (Coumadin) for example, is sometimes prescribed for people who have had a TIA or ischemic stroke, and for people with certain heart conditions or other conditions associated with increased blood clottings. The effectiveness of this blood-thinning medication can be altered by certain foods, supplements, and medications. The key is to be consistent in eating certain foods and to be careful with certain drug combinations.

Vitamin K counteracts anticoagulants, increasing the necessary dose. Although you should avoid taking supplements that contain vitamin K, you may eat foods containing the vitamin if you eat about the same amount each day. These foods include the following:

Asparagus
Avocado
Beans w/pod, raw

Broccoli

Brussels sprouts

Cabbage

Cauliflower

Coleslaw

Collard greens

Cucumber, raw, unpeeled

Endive

Garbanzo beans (chickpeas)

Green scallion

Kale

Lentils

Lettuce

Liver (beef, pork, chicken)

Mustard greens, raw

Parsley

Peas (green)

Pickle, dill

Sauerkraut

Seaweed

Soybeans

Spinach

Swiss chard

Turnip greens

Watercress

Chewing tobacco also contains a high amount of vitamin K.

Other foods, beverages, and herbal supplements can also affect anticoagulant therapy and should be consumed in consistent amounts. These include the following:

Canola, salad, olive, and soybean oils

Mayonnaise

Margarine

Alcoholic beverages (limit yourself to no more than two
  drinks per day)
Green tea (a light color tea whose leaves have not been
  completely fermented)
Sweet Clover/Woodruff tea
Danshen (an herb)
Devil's Claw (an herb)
Dong Quai (an herb)
Papain (a component of unripened pineapple that is used
  in meat tenderizer and medicines)

Certain medications, as well as an alteration of dosage, can also affect the way anticoagulants work. Let your doctor know what medications you are taking and at what dosage. Notify him or her about any changes in your medications. Notify all members of your health care team that you are taking an anticoagulant. And check with your doctor or pharmacist before using nonprescription drugs.

Medications that may interact with or alter the effectiveness of anticoagulant therapy include the following:

Nonprescription medications like cold or cough
  preparations, antacids, laxatives, and vitamins
Aspirin
Nonsteroidal anti-inflammatory medications such as
  ibuprofen and naproxen
Long-term acetaminophen
Amiodarone (Cordarone)
Cimetidine (Tagamet)
Erythromycin
Omeprazole (Prilosec)
Tamoxifen (Nolvadex)
Trimethoprim-sulfamethoxazole (Bactrim, Septra)

Antiplatelet Agents

Antiplatelet agents thin the blood, though in a much less profound way than anticoagulants. The most well known of these drugs is aspirin, which is inexpensive, relatively safe, and extremely familiar. Other, newer drugs in the class include clopidogrel (Plavix), a combination of dipyridamole and aspirin (Aggrenox), and ticlopidine (Ticlid). These medications, like anticoagulants, can play an important role in the treatment of such conditions as ischemic heart disease and ischemic stroke. Antiplatelet agents, like anticoagulants, carry the risk of causing intracerebral hemorrhage. Theoretically, antiplatelet agents, or platelet inhibitors, may also increase the risk of hemorrhage in people with intracranial aneurysms or vascular malformations. If you have any other risk factors for hemorrhagic stroke, you may want to talk with your doctor about the risk conveyed by antiplatelet agents. He or she may be able to make a recommendation for an alternative medication. In addition, you should consider using acetaminophen (Tylenol) instead of aspirin for pain relief and fever reduction.

Arteritis

Arteritis is an inflammation of the arteries. It can affect arteries anywhere in the body, including in the vessels of the brain. As you might expect, this can lead to ischemic stroke. Arteritis also slightly increases the risk of intracerebral hemorrhage and subarachnoid hemorrhage. Reducing this risk requires reducing the inflammation. This is usually done with medications.

MEDICAL

The choice of medication for arteritis depends on its cause. Some cases are caused by such inflammatory conditions as systemic lupus erythematosus; others are caused by infection. Noninfectious arteritis is generally treated with anti-inflammatory medications like corticosteroids; infectious arteritis is generally treated with antimicrobial medications.

Anti-inflammatory Medications

Conditions that can cause arteritis include lupus, polyarteritis nodosa, giant-cell angiitis, Takayasu's arteritis, Behçet's disease, and, in rare cases, rheumatoid arteritis and Sjögren's syndrome. Treatment for these conditions varies greatly. In most cases, the arteritis that results is treated in a similar manner: with anti-inflammatory medications like corticosteroids. The most commonly prescribed steroid is prednisone, which along with other steroid medications is related to hormones produced by the adrenal glands. They can reduce swelling and inflammation rapidly, but steroids are not without side effects. Given in large doses for a long period of time, steroids can cause weight gain, bone loss, muscle wasting, blurred vision, cataracts, a reduced resistance to infection, and increased blood pressure. In addition, they cause the body to cease producing its own natural steroids. For this reason, you cannot simply quit taking steroids all at once. You have to taper off gradually to allow your body time to resume normal steroid production. When anti-inflammatory medications do not work on their own, they may be combined with such immunosuppressive medications as cyclophosphamide or azathioprine.

Antimicrobials

Infectious arteritis can be caused by any of a variety of bacteria, viruses, and fungi as well as by bacterial endocarditis if it causes an embolism that makes its way to the brain. The choice of medication depends, obviously, on the type of infection and the type of organism that's causing it. Among the infections that can cause arteritis are bacterial infections like syphilis and malaria; viral infections, herpes simplex and herpes zoster for example; and fungal infections including aspergillosis and candida. For such bacterial infections as meningitis, an inflammation of the membranes that line the brain and spinal cord, the choice is generally an antibiotic. The actual bacteria will dictate the appropriate antibiotic. For example, penicillin may be administered if the infection is caused by pneumococcus, while nafcillin, oxacillin, or methicillin may be administered if *Staphylococcus aureus* is the culprit. This is because certain antibiotics are more effective than others at killing certain organisms. Fungal infections, for their part, are treated by such medications as amphotericin B and flucytosine. Viral infections are more difficult to treat, but the recent development of medications like acyclovir makes treatment feasible.

One thing that should be noted about infectious arteritis: people who have transient ischemic attacks or minor ischemic strokes in conjunction with this inflammatory condition generally are not treated with anticoagulant medications as are most other people with TIA, because infectious arteritis can trigger hemorrhage. For this reason, treatment generally focuses on eradicating the infection.

Artery Blockage or Narrowing (Stenosis)

If you've been diagnosed with an artery blockage or stenosis in one of your carotid or coronary arteries, you probably have atherosclerosis. Stroke prevention, for you, will likely focus on opening up the affected artery to improve blood flow and slowing or stopping the progression of atherosclerosis. The latter is addressed the same way regardless of where the blockage is; the former is not. In this section, I address stenosis or blockage of the intracranial arteries and the carotid arteries. (I address coronary artery blockage in the "Ischemic Heart Disease" section on page 155.)

Carotid artery stenosis is a leading cause of transient ischemic attack and minor ischemic stroke, which are essentially its primary symptoms. These symptoms can also be caused by a blockage of one of the other arteries that supply the brain, including the vertebral arteries and the basilar artery. If you have experienced either of these symptoms, refer to the "Transient Ischemic Attack/Minor Ischemic Stroke" section on page 175 for a rundown of the treatments available and the efforts you can take to prevent a future ischemic stroke. Not all instances of intracranial artery stenosis—or even complete blockage, or occlusion—produce these symptoms, however. You may have been diagnosed with carotid artery stenosis based on the results of a neurologic exam or imaging test performed for some other reason, or because your doctor detected a swishing sound, called a bruit, when he or she listened to your neck with a stethoscope. If this is the case, your treatment options—most notably your surgical options—may differ from those listed in the "Transient Ischemic Attack/Minor Ischemic Stroke" section.

SURGICAL/INTERVENTIONAL

Generally speaking, the surgical options for asymptomatic narrowing or blockage of the carotid artery are the same as those for TIA or minor ischemic stroke: carotid endarterectomy, carotid angioplasty, and artery-artery bypass. If the blockage or narrowing has not produced symptoms, you are much less likely to undergo any of these procedures. The primary determining factor in whether or not you should be a candidate for surgery is the degree to which your artery is narrowed or blocked. A secondary factor is the presence of ulcers, clots, or complex lesions in the artery.

Carotid Endarterectomy

This procedure, in which the surgeon makes an incision in the neck, clamps off the carotid artery, opens the artery, scrapes off the atherosclerotic plaque on the artery's inner lining, then closes the artery and removes the clamps, can significantly reduce ischemic stroke risk in certain people—most notably those who experience such symptoms as TIA and who have significant narrowing in one or both of their carotid arteries. It is generally not recommended for people with a complete carotid artery blockage, or occlusion, because occlusions often extend through a large portion of the artery, making surgery technically unfeasible. In addition, occluded arteries often harbor embedded clots that could be released during surgery and cause ischemic stroke. In people with less significant narrowing who don't experience symptoms, the procedure can have little or no effect on ischemic stroke risk. What's more, even among these people, the procedure has the potential to trigger ischemic stroke and heart attack and, rarely, hemorrhagic stroke. Other surgical complications, including reaction to the anesthetic, infection, and scarring, are also possible. You and your doctor must seriously consider these risks—as well as the potential benefits of the procedure—before you decide on this option.

Although the procedure can theoretically be performed on anyone who has stenosis, or narrowing, of one or both of the carotid arteries, it is most beneficial for patients who have experienced symptoms like TIA and who have a significant reduction in the diameter of the corresponding carotid artery. In some cases, the reduction alone warrants the procedure. Studies indicate that people with a stenosis that reduces the diameter of the artery by 60 percent or more may benefit from the procedure even if they do not have symptoms—as long as they are otherwise healthy and are not considered poor surgical risks. This is particularly true of people who have visible ulcers, clots, or complex lesions on the artery. In people who fit these criteria, the procedure can reduce ischemic stroke caused by the artery in question from about 2 percent a year over five years to a rate of about 1 percent a year, although men are more likely to benefit than women. The procedure is generally not performed for symptom-free people whose blockage reduces the diameter of

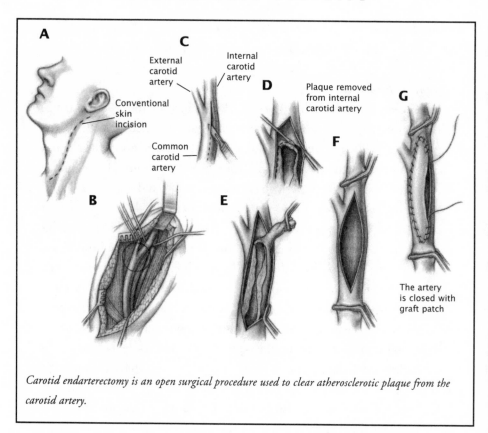

A

C

External carotid artery

Internal carotid artery

D

Plaque removed from internal carotid artery

G

Conventional skin incision

Common carotid artery

F

B

E

The artery is closed with graft patch

Carotid endarterectomy is an open surgical procedure used to clear atherosclerotic plaque from the carotid artery.

the carotid artery by less than 60 percent or for people with blockages of 60 percent or more who are considered moderate or high surgical risks.

Since carotid endarterectomy conveys risk, it should be performed only by an experienced surgeon with a low rate of complications and death. If you opt for this procedure, I recommend that you find a surgeon with a combined complication and death rate for the procedure of less than 6 percent on patients with symptoms and less than 3 percent on patients without symptoms. These rates are often difficult to determine accurately, in large part because some surgeons may not have performed the procedure often enough to ensure statistical validity.

Carotid Artery Angioplasty

Another surgical option for treating a carotid artery blockage and reducing the risk of major ischemic stroke is carotid angioplasty. Although this procedure, in which a balloon-tipped catheter is threaded through the blood vessels into the blocked carotid artery, then inflated to open the artery and facilitate blood flow, is being used in some medical centers, it is still considered experimental. Its effectiveness has not yet been adequately compared to that of carotid endarterectomy, and nobody knows in what instances it will prove to be preferable. That said, the procedure does have some apparent advantages—including local, rather than general anesthesia, the lack of an incision and, generally, an expectation of a shorter recovery period and hospital stay. There are some instances when it might be considered: for example, if you have a condition that increases the risk of open surgery, but you are otherwise a candidate for carotid endarterectomy, or if the technical aspect of approaching the artery in an open procedure is extremely difficult. Carotid angioplasty is not without potential complications. The procedure can result in dissection or rupture of the carotid artery or the formation of an aneurysm, embolism, or blood vessel blockage. At this point, carotid angioplasty is not widely recommended or widely available. Angioplasty may also be performed on blockages in other intracranial arteries, although again, the procedure is not widespread.

Extracranial-Intracranial Bypass

Another surgical option available for people with a blockage or narrowing of the carotid artery or another intracranial artery is extracranial-to-intracranial bypass. This procedure, which involves the diversion of blood from one of the external arteries supplying structures outside the skull to an internal artery, was once widely performed to prevent ischemic stroke, but the results of a major study published in 1985 found that it is generally ineffective as a stroke preventive. There are some rare instances when this procedure may be useful. If a large aneurysm or tumor is blocking or invading an artery, for example, the sacrifice of the artery may help prevent ischemic stroke. The procedure may also be recommended if a blockage or high-grade narrowing of an artery is causing repeated, incapacitating TIAs or progressive visual loss.

MEDICAL

Medication, in the form of anticoagulants and antiplatelet agents, is a standard stroke preventive for people with narrowing or blockage of the carotid artery or another intracranial artery, like the vertebral artery or the basilar artery. The choice of medications depends largely on whether or not the narrowing or blockage produces symptoms. If you've experienced a TIA or similar event, your options include anticoagulants as well as antiplatelet agents (see "Transient Ischemic Attack/Minor Ischemic Stroke" on page 175). If you have been diagnosed with a blockage but have no symptoms, you are more likely to be treated with antiplatelet agents—alone or in combination with carotid endarterectomy. These medications include aspirin, clopidogrel (Plavix), Aggrenox (a combination of dipyridamole and aspirin), and ticlopidine (Ticlid). They are considered standard treatment for asymptomatic carotid stenosis, although their effectiveness in reducing ischemic stroke risk is less certain. They may also help reduce the risk of heart attack, another condition related to underlying atherosclerotic disease.

Depending on your personal situation, medical treatment may also include drugs to treat diabetes and/or hypertension. These conditions commonly occur in conjunction with atherosclerosis and are known to exacerbate it.

LIFESTYLE

Lifestyle changes that address the development and progression of atherosclerosis—the underlying cause of most instances of artery narrowing—are among the best ways to treat carotid artery stenosis or stenosis of another intracranial artery. Unlike the other treatments I discuss, they target atherosclerosis all over the body, and they do it in a natural way. Every medication and surgical procedure has some side effect or risk, but such lifestyle changes as diet, smoking, and stress reduction do not. In fact, they offer health benefits other than simply treating atherosclerosis. I strongly recommend that you opt for these changes when you design your prescription, regardless of the medical or surgical treatments you choose.

Diet

A diet high in fat and cholesterol leads to the development of atherosclerotic plaque in the arteries. If you have been diagnosed with a blockage or narrowing of one or both of your carotid arteries, chances are good that it is atherosclerosis, and you already have a buildup. To stop this buildup from progressing—and potentially even reverse it—you should eat a diet that is very low in saturated fat and cholesterol. Research among people with atherosclerosis of the coronary arteries indicates that atherosclerosis can be stopped or reversed with a diet that restricts fat intake to less than 10 percent of total calories and cholesterol intake to less than 5 milligrams per day. Although studies have not yet indicated whether such a diet can reverse atherosclerotic buildup in the carotid arteries, I believe it makes sense to reduce saturated fat and cholesterol intake to a level somewhat comparable to that. The typical American gets approximately 40 percent of his or her calories from fat and takes in 400 milligrams of cholesterol a day. If you are really serious about treating—or reversing—atherosclerosis, you have to do much more than follow the "healthy diet" guidelines recommended by the federal government and many health organizations. These guidelines, which restrict fat intake to no more than 30 percent of total calories and cholesterol intake to no more than 300 milligrams of cholesterol a day, are simply ineffective. I believe we need to go further. I discuss my dietary recommendations in detail in the next chapter.

Smoking Cessation

Like diet, smoking contributes to the development and progression of atherosclerosis. If you have been diagnosed with carotid stenosis, there's a good chance that you already have atherosclerosis. If you smoke, you help the disease progress and increase your risk of having a major ischemic stroke. Regardless of the treatment option or options that you choose, you should seriously consider smoking cessation. I discuss various methods to help you quit on page 169. You should also avoid passive smoke.

Stress Reduction

The link between stress and atherosclerosis is an indirect one, but I believe stress reduction plays a role in bringing atherosclerosis under control—or preventing its development. Stress is known to increase blood pressure, and high blood pressure has been linked to atherosclerosis. In fact, the two often go hand in hand. For suggestions on how to decrease your stress level, see page 174 and chapter 5.

Atrial Fibrillation

Atrial fibrillation is a relatively common cause of cardioembolic ischemic stroke; it is also the most common chronic heart arrhythmia in the United

States, affecting approximately 2.2 million people. Fortunately, treatment of this condition can reduce stroke risk. Perhaps even more exciting, we are on the verge of predicting who will develop atrial fibrillation and, possibly, treating those people to prevent the condition from developing. This, obviously, would have a significant impact on stroke risk and incidence. Atrial fibrillation is responsible for an estimated 75,000 strokes in the United States each year. You can read more about this development in chapters 5 and 8. Here, I discuss what can be done if you've already been diagnosed with the condition. The options range from cardioversion, an interventional technique, to medications to control heart rhythm or to prevent clot formation.

INTERVENTIONAL

If you have recently been diagnosed with atrial fibrillation, your doctor may recommend cardioversion. If you're a fan of TV medical dramas, you've probably seen this shock treatment procedure performed when a patient has flatlined (his or her heart has stopped beating). In this treatment, synchronized electrical shock is delivered to the heart by means of two metal paddles placed on a person's chest. The procedure is designed to restore the heart to its normal rhythm. It does this by momentarily stopping the heart—and the irregular rhythm. Cardioversion is generally performed under a short-acting general anesthetic. Since the shock has the potential to generate or release clots, particularly in people who have a history of clots, an enlarged heart, congestive heart failure, or valvular heart disease, you will likely be treated with an anticoagulant like warfarin for several weeks before the procedure is performed. Generally, cardioversion is most successful in restoring normal rhythm if atrial fibrillation has only recently occurred. Long-term, or chronic, atrial fibrillation is usually treated with medications.

MEDICAL

Medical treatment for atrial fibrillation may include antiarrhythmic medications, which alter the way in which the electrical current flows through the heart and alter the heart rhythm; digitalis, which is prescribed if atrial fibrillation is accompanied by rapid ventricular response (a rapid beating of the ventricles, or lower chambers of the heart); and anticoagulants or antiplatelet agents to prevent the development of clots. Antihypertensive medications, too, may play a role in atrial fibrillation.

Antiarrhythmic Agents

These medications, which include quinidine (Cardioquin, Cin-quin, Dura-quin, Quinaglute, Quinalan, Quinidex, Quinora), procainamide (Procan SR, Pronestyl), disopyramide (Norpace), lidocaine (Xylocaine), phenytoin (Dilantin), mexiletine (Mexitil), tocainimide (Tonocard), flecainide (Tambocor), moricizine (Ethmozine), and propafenone (Rythmol), may be used to control symptoms of atrial fibrillation if the symptoms are severe and do not respond to cardioversion. Studies have shown that antiarrhythmic drugs should be avoided if possible and used with caution when necessary. This is because all of the medications can cause potentially significant side effects. In fact, they can actually provoke heart rhythm disorders. For this reason, your doctor will want to make sure that there is a good reason to prescribe one of these medications and will want to monitor you while you are taking the drug. Fortunately, several antihypertensive medications can have normalizing effects on heart rhythm. Since these medications carry fewer side effects than traditional antiarrhythmic agents, your doctor may prescribe one of them instead.

Anticoagulants and Antiplatelets

Anticoagulants are mainstays of atrial fibrillation treatment—particularly when it comes to stroke prevention. These medications, the most commonly prescribed of which is warfarin (Coumadin), thin the blood and reduce the risk of clot formation. Warfarin is generally prescribed as a long-term treatment. It is particularly helpful in reducing ischemic stroke in people with atrial fibrillation who have had a transient ischemic attack or minor ischemic stroke within the previous two years. The primary side effect of warfarin and other anticoagulants is bleeding or hemorrhage. People at risk of hemorrhage may take aspirin or another antiplatelet agent if they cannot take an anticoagulant. These medications also thin the blood, but less effectively; consequently, they carry less risk of causing bleeding.

Antihypertensives

Antihypertensives, beta-blockers and calcium channel blockers for example, may play a role in the treatment of atrial fibrillation. Such beta-blockers as propranolol (Inderal), Nadolol (Corgard), and atenolol (Tenormin) and such calcium channel blockers as verapamil (Calan, Isoptin, Verelan) can help slow or normalize certain fast heart rhythms. This makes them ideal for treating people with both atrial fibrillation and hypertension. They also may be used to treat either condition individually. Angiotensin II inhibitors, ACE inhibitors, and beta-blockers may attack atrial fibrillation on another front. These antihypertensive medications appear to help treat endothelial dysfunction, which may be an underlying cause of atrial fibrillation. I discuss the risks and benefits of these medications in the "Hypertension" section.

Bleeding Disorders

Bleeding disorders like hemophilia and blood conditions that promote bleeding like thrombocytopenia (a low level of blood platelets) and low prothrombin (a component in blood that causes it to clot) can cause hemorrhagic stroke. Treatment depends on the condition itself and the condition of the person. Thrombocytopenia, for example, is often treated with transfusions of platelets. In severe cases, a bone marrow transplant may be in order to help the body produce more platelets. Low prothrombin is generally treated with fresh frozen plasma and/or vitamin K, which helps the blood to clot. Hemophilia is treated by replacing clotting factor VIII or clotting factor IX, components of the blood that are deficient in people with the disease.

Body Mass Index

Body mass index (BMI), a measurement of weight per unit of height, is a better indicator of body fat and a better predictor of health than weight alone. The medical community uses this measurement to determine if a person is overweight or underweight. Overall there is a tendency for people with an increased BMI (greater than or equal to 25) to have a greater risk of ischemic stroke. This is largely because being overweight places you at risk for high blood pressure, ischemic heart disease, diabetes mellitus, and high total and LDL cholesterol levels. It can also increase triglyceride levels and lower HDL cholesterol levels. All of these factors can increase your risk of ischemic stroke. For reasons that are less clear, being underweight (BMI less than 19) appears to slightly increase the risk of subarachnoid hemorrhage. To reduce your stroke risk, you should aim for a BMI of 19 to 24. Depending on your situation, this involves either losing or gaining weight.

Weight is a combination of several factors, including your genetics (which play a part in how you metabolize food), how much and what you eat, and how much you exercise. Obviously, the most natural and healthy way to lose or gain weight is to change your eating and exercise habits. The formula is simple in theory: to lose weight, you need to eat less and exercise more; to gain weight, you need to eat more and/or exercise less. In reality, it's not that simple. Fasting, skipping meals, or otherwise severely restricting your food intake can lead to nutritional deficiencies and be unhealthy. Likewise, adopting a sedentary lifestyle in an effort to gain weight deprives the body of the health benefits of exercise. In some cases, other factors also come into play. Eating disorders like anorexia nervosa and bulimia and conditions that affect the metabolism like hypo- or hyperthyroidism can alter the basic formula.

If one of these underlying conditions is responsible for your weight problem, you will need to work with your doctor to treat it. You may also need to work with your doctor if you are extremely overweight or have been unsuccessful in changing your diet and exercise patterns. Although these lifestyle factors are the mainstay of weight control, surgical procedures and medications are available for people who fit certain criteria. In addition, your doctor may be able to help you change your diet and adopt an exercise program you can live with.

Since being overweight poses more health disadvantages than being underweight and since the eating disorders that are responsible for some people being underweight are beyond the scope of this book, I detail only the methods and treatments for weight loss. If you are mildly underweight and are at risk for atherosclerotic ischemic stroke or any other type of ischemic stroke, you don't need to worry about your weight from a standpoint of stroke prevention. If you are underweight and have other risk factors for subarachnoid hemorrhage, you should consider taking measures to put on a little weight. Enjoy the opportunity to eat a little bit more. Just make sure to choose healthy foods. Needing to gain weight is not an invitation to eat high-fat, high-cholesterol foods, which can cause other health problems.

SURGICAL/INTERVENTIONAL

Several surgical procedures can be used to treat overweight individuals, although they should be used with extreme caution and as last resorts. These procedures, known as bariatric surgical procedures, are generally recommended only for people who are morbidly obese (a BMI of 40 or more). These procedures are drastic measures that alter the digestive system and can cause numerous gastrointestinal side effects. They generally follow one of two basic approaches.

Malabsorptive procedures are designed to decrease the amount of food absorbed. These procedures include constructing a pouch that bypasses much of the stomach and some of the small intestine. Potential side effects include surgical complications, vitamin deficiencies, and gastrointestinal distress.

Restrictive surgical procedures decrease the amount of food a person can ingest. This can be done using staples or a band to reduce the size of the stomach. Potential side effects include surgical complications and staple erosion, which can lead to weight gain. In fact, long-term maintenance of weight loss for any of the available surgical procedures remains under study.

MEDICATIONS

As much as many of us would love to be able to eat as much as we want, then take a pill to keep us slender, no such magic pill has been invented, and some of our attempts have had somewhat frightening results. Redux and one of the two prescription medications in the "fen-phen" combination that was popularly prescribed in the late 1990s, for example, were pulled off the market in 1997 because they were linked to heart valve problems. That's not to say that other medications have no role in weight loss in certain cases. They just don't have solo—or even preferred—status. A number of medications have been found to boost weight loss by about 5 to 10 percent, but only when they are used in conjunction with diet and exercise. These medications carry the potential risk of side effects, and weight may return when they are discontinued.

Amphetamine-like Drugs

The majority of medications prescribed to enhance weight loss are molecularly similar to the amphetamines, a class of stimulant drugs that suppress appetite but are highly addictive. These drugs, which include mazindol (Mazanor, Sanorex); phendimetrazine (Bontril, Plegine, Adipost, Dital, Dyrexan, Melfiat, Prelu-2, Rexigen Forte); benzphetamine (Didrex); and phentermine (Fastin, Ionamin) suppress the appetite, stimulate the central nervous system, and may have other metabolic effects. Phenylpropanolamine (Dextrim, Acutrim), a nonprescription weight-loss medication, was taken off the market in late 2000 because of concerns about increased risk of hemorrhagic stroke. In studies, obese individuals who take these drugs and follow a low-calorie diet lose weight slightly faster than those who lose weight on diet alone, but the difference is typically only a fraction of a pound per week and decreases over time. In addition, these medications carry the risk of side effects, including nervousness, irritability, insomnia, increased blood pressure, heart palpitations, nausea, constipation, and dry mouth.

Sibutramine (Meridia)

One of the newest weight-loss drugs on the market, sibutramine, inhibits the reuptake of the brain chemicals serotonin and norepinephrine. It has been found to limit both appetite and food intake, when used in conjunction with a reduced-calorie diet and exercise. Sibutramine is not recommended for people with a BMI less than 30, unless other health problems warrant immediate medical intervention. Its most common side effects are constipation, headache, insomnia, and dry mouth. It can also cause a slight increase in blood pressure.

Orlistat (Xenical)

Orlistat, approved by the U.S. Food and Drug Administration (FDA) in 1999, aids weight loss by cutting the amount of fat the body absorbs by about 30 percent. The unabsorbed fat is eliminated in the stool, which can result in such side effects as oily spotting, gas with discharge, an urgent need to defecate, oily or fatty stools, increased bowel movements, and an inability to control bowel movements. Studies indicate that side effects usually improve with a decrease in dietary fat. Since the medication reduces the absorption of fat, it may affect your absorption of fat-soluble vitamins, vitamins A, D, E, and K. Other potential side effects include abdominal pain and nausea. The FDA recommends that people taking orlistat take vitamin supplements containing these vitamins two hours before taking the drug.

Fluoxetine (Prozac)

Although Prozac is an antidepressant, it has been found to help some people lose weight. It has been suggested that the mechanisms by which it does this include treating depression (which sometimes results in weight gain), inhibiting appetite, or increasing metabolism. For more information about Prozac, see the "Depression" section on page 131.

LIFESTYLE

Diet and exercise are the key to weight loss. Food is the body's energy source. Your body burns food to produce energy. The amount of energy in food is measured by kilocalories, or calories. When you take in 3,500 calories, you gain a pound. When you burn off 3,500 calories, you lose a pound. To lose weight, you must take in fewer calories than you burn off. This generally means either eating less, exercising more, or a combination of the two. Generally speaking, the combination is more effective.

Diet

The amount of calories you need to maintain your weight is determined by your weight and activity level. To lose weight through diet, you need to choose foods wisely that allow you to eat as much as you want but take in fewer calories. The amount of calories you cut (along with the amount of exercise you add) will determine the rate at which you will lose weight. For example, if you cut 500 calories a day from your diet, in one week (seven days), you will lose one pound. Rather than fasting, skipping meals, or severely restricting your food intake to cut your calories, make wise food choices. Choose foods that are low in fat and low in calories. That way you can eat as much as you want. When you fast or skip meals, you may miss getting important nutrients. You may also slow your metabolism and lose control of your appetite, which could result in your eating more later.

Try to eat a balanced, low-fat, low-calorie diet. Fat is not only a contributor to atherosclerosis, it is a contributor to obesity. Each gram of fat contains nine calories. Carbohydrates and protein, on the other hand, contain only four calories per gram. So a high-fat diet tends to be higher in calories. In addition, although the body uses carbohydrates quite rapidly, it tends to store fats, which can lead to weight gain.

See chapter 5 for my dietary recommendations. Although my diet is designed to prevent stroke rather than promote weight loss, many of my patients have lost weight on the program. If weight loss is your goal, pay

attention to your calorie intake as well as your fat, saturated fat, and cholesterol intake.

Exercise

Exercise is the other major component of weight loss. Every time you exercise, you burn off calories, and the more calories you burn off, the more
weight you will lose. For exercise to have a real effect on your weight, you
need to do it regularly: at least thirty minutes three or more times a week. I
outline a number of exercise recommendations in chapter 5.

Cardiomyopathy

Cardiomyopathy affects about 50,000 Americans, far fewer than ischemic
heart disease, yet it is a leading cause of heart transplantation. This disorder
of the heart muscle is serious by itself, and it can lead to congestive heart
failure, arrhythmias, and many other problems, as well as to cardioembolic
ischemic stroke. Treatment for cardiomyopathy depends on its type, cause,
and severity. It can range from bed rest to reduce strain on the heart, to
medications to ease the strain on the heart, to surgery to relieve symptoms,
to heart transplant.

SURGICAL

Heart transplantation is the most extreme of the surgical procedures used to
treat cardiomyopathy. It is generally reserved for people in whom cardiomyopathy has caused congestive heart failure and weakened the heart to
the point that it no longer responds to medication. Even with those restrictions, not all people will qualify. A limited number of donor hearts are available, so doctors take into consideration such other factors as your age,
health, and willingness to comply with medical recommendations to determine if you are among those most likely to benefit from the procedure. I
discuss the procedure in more detail in the "Congestive Heart Failure" section on page 128.

If you have hypertrophic cardiomyopathy, the type in which the heart
muscle becomes overgrown, you may be a candidate for a surgical procedure known as myotomy-myectomy. This procedure is generally recommended only when the overgrowth obstructs blood flow. It involves

removing the portion of overgrown heart muscle that is causing the blockage. It can effectively relieve some symptoms, but it carries risks.

MEDICAL

Medications are mainstays of cardiomyopathy treatment, particularly when it comes to preventing ischemic stroke. These drugs include positive inotropic medications, which strengthen the heart's contraction, and diuretics, which reduce fluid accumulation, as well as anticoagulants or antiplatelet agents, if clotting is a problem. Other medications may also be used if congestive heart failure is present. These medications are detailed in the "Congestive Heart Failure" section.

Positive Inotropic Medications

These medications are designed to strengthen the heart's contraction strength. The most well known of these medications is digitalis, which has been used to treat heart problems for more than two hundred years. Digitalis and such related medications as digoxin (Lanoxin) increase the pumping strength of the heart and can help control certain rhythm disorders. Studies indicate that digitalis can help improve symptoms and reduce hospitalization, although it has little or no effect on survival. Potential side effects include slow or irregular heartbeat, visual disturbances, loss of appetite, and stomach upset.

Diuretics

Diuretics help eliminate excess fluid from the body. Cardiomyopathy can lead to fluid accumulation in the legs, abdomen, liver, and lungs, so these common antihypertensive medications can play a role in its treatment. I describe these drugs in more detail in the "Hypertension" section on page 139.

Anticoagulants and Antiplatelets

Not all people with cardiomyopathy require treatment with anticoagulants, but some may benefit, particularly those whose condition has resulted in clot formation. These drugs thin the blood, making it flow more easily and reducing the risk of clot formation. The most commonly prescribed anticoagulant is warfarin (Coumadin). Its primary side effect is bleeding or hemorrhage. When a bleeding condition or some other condition makes anti-coagulants inadvisable, such antiplatelet agents as aspirin or clopidogrel (Plavix) can be used.

LIFESTYLE
In addition to medication to treat cardiomyopathy and reduce the risk of ischemic stroke, your doctor may recommend bed rest, to reduce your heart's workload, and a reduction of sodium intake. Sodium causes the body to retain water and usually has a detrimental effect on blood pressure. You may also be advised to reduce your stress level.

Cholesterol and Triglyceride Levels
High blood cholesterol levels, particularly high blood levels of total choles-terol and low-density lipoprotein (LDL), the so-called bad cholesterol, increase the risk of atherosclerosis, which, as you know, increases the risk of ischemic stroke. High levels of triglycerides, too, affect ischemic stroke risk. Reducing cholesterol and triglyceride levels would seem to reduce the risk of ischemic stroke. Research has not yet conclusively proved this to be true, largely, I suspect, because studies have not examined cholesterol's effects on the various subtypes of stroke. If your total cholesterol is above 200 mg/dL and/or your LDL level is above 130 mg/dL, or your triglyceride level is above 200 mg/dL, you should consider lowering them (150 mg/dL is a good level to aspire to for total cholesterol; 90 mg/dL for LDL). This can be particularly beneficial if you have atherosclerosis or other risk factors for atherosclerotic ischemic stroke, including a family history of the condition. The healthiest way to lower your cholesterol and triglycerides, in my opinion, is by means of diet, exercise, and stress reduction. Medications and food additives are available if you cannot achieve your target goal by lifestyle changes alone.

MEDICAL
Several classes of cholesterol-lowering medications are on the market, and new drugs are appearing regularly. Also growing is the number of foods and food additives, including margarines and salad dressings, that are designed to reduce cholesterol levels. These medications and food additives have their place in controlling cholesterol, but they do not stand alone. They are meant to be used in addition to—not in place of—diet, exercise, and stress

reduction. I don't believe medications should be the first line of treatment. They may be added to your treatment regimen more quickly if your cholesterol level is extremely high and you have heart disease or other risk factors for heart disease and ischemic stroke. Generally speaking, medications are not recommended unless your LDL level is 130 mg/dL or greater and you have been diagnosed with heart disease, your LDL level is 160 mg/dL or more and you have two or more other risk factors for heart disease, or your LDL number is 190 mg/dL and you have fewer than two other risk factors for heart disease. This does not mean that you must start on medication if you fit one of these conditions. These are just guidelines for the points at which medications are often recommended. It is possible to significantly reduce even high cholesterol levels without medications. I have personally seen people reduce their total cholesterol level from 600 to 150 mg/dL with lifestyle modifications alone.

If you and your doctor decide that lipid-lowering medication should be included in your stroke prevention prescription, you will have to consider the various types of medications out there and choose the one that best meets your needs. The various classes of lipid-lowering drugs work in different ways and have different effects.

Bile Acid Binding Resins

These medications, which include cholestyramine (Questran, Prevalite) and colestipol (Colestid), prevent cholesterol from being absorbed in the body and promote its excretion. This reduces stores of cholesterol in the liver and causes the liver to draw in more cholesterol from the blood, which reduces blood cholesterol levels. Bile acid binding resins can reduce LDL cholesterol levels by 15 to 25 percent, depending on how high the level is to start. These medications are a common first choice for people who need that level of LDL reduction, because they seldom cause serious side effects. This is because they are not actually absorbed into the body. Their most common side effect is constipation, which may be relieved by a psyllium-based laxative. Other side effects include abdominal pain and stomach upset, including nausea, belching, and bloating. Since these drugs may also interfere with the absorption of other medications, you should take other medications one hour before or four to six hours after.

Statin Drugs

Officially known as HMG CoA reductase inhibitors, these drugs, the chemical names of which end in-*statin,* are among the most commonly prescribed lipid medications, because they can have a positive effect on multiple lipid levels: total cholesterol, LDL cholesterol, triglycerides, and high-density lipoprotein (HDL), the so-called good cholesterol. HDL escorts cholesterol out of the body, lowering LDL and total cholesterol levels. Statins work by blocking the production of cholesterol in the liver, which causes the organ to take more in from the blood. Depending on the drug, the dose, and your cholesterol level, these drugs can reduce total and LDL cholesterol levels by 20 to 30 percent. They can also reduce triglycerides by 7 to 20 percent and increase HDL levels by 6 to 12 percent. Statin drugs include atorvastatin (Lipitor), lovastatin (Mevacor), pravastatin (Pravachol), simvastatin (Zocor), cerivastatin (Baycol), and fluvastatin (Lescol). All have relatively similar side effects. Since the most serious is liver function problems, you may be requested to undergo regular liver function tests after you start taking one of these medications. Other potential side effects include muscle pain and weakness (the risk is increased when the drug is combined with the lipid-lowering drugs gemfibrozil and nicotinic acid or with the antibiotics erythromycin and cyclosporin), blurred vision, stomach upset, insomnia, and headache.

Fibric Acid Derivatives

These drugs, which include gemfibrozil (Lopid), clofibrate (Atromid-S), and fenofibrate (Tricor), help the liver break down very-low-density lipoprotein, which causes LDL and triglyceride levels to drop and HDL levels to increase. The way they do this is not well understood. They are generally prescribed for people who have very high triglyceride levels. Side effects of these drugs can be serious. They include gallstones, kidney problems, liver function problems, stomach upset, muscle pain and weakness, dizziness, and blurred vision.

Nicotinic Acid

This drug, a form of the B vitamin niacin, reduces the body's ability to manufacture very-low-density lipoprotein (VLDL), which the body converts into LDL cholesterol. Ultimately, it reduces both LDL and triglyceride levels. In people with cholesterol levels of 240 mg/dL or higher, it could reduce total cholesterol and LDL cholesterol levels by 10 to 20 percent. It also increases levels of HDL an average of 20 to 35 percent. The most common side effect is a temporary, warm, flushing sensation that usually occurs on the face and upper body. Other possible side effects include headache, stomach upset, and itching. The most serious side effect is liver function problems. Side effects can be minimized somewhat by starting the drug at a low dose and building up to a recommended dose. They can also be reduced by taking the drug with food. Although nicotinic acid is found in some foods, supplementation is required to achieve cholesterol-lowering effects. The supplement is available over the counter, but it should not be used without medical supervision. Prescription varieties are also available. Some brand names include Nia-Bid, Niacels, Nicobid, Nicolar, Sl-Niacin, and Nicotinix.

Probucol

Sold under the brand name Lorelco, probucol is generally prescribed only to people who have not responded well to other lipid-lowering drugs. The drug, which operates differently from the other medications, can reduce LDL cholesterol by 10 to 20 percent, but it also can decrease HDL cholesterol by 10 to 30 percent. It has no effect on triglycerides. Potential side effects include stomach upset, diarrhea, insomnia, and more serious conditions including irregular heartbeat and gastrointestinal bleeding.

Foods and Food Additives

Some foods and food additives have a pharmacological effect. They are sold in the grocery store and do not require a prescription. At this point, they consist primarily of margarines, Benecol and Take Control, for example, and a number of salad dressings, although I have no doubt that the variety will grow. These foods are designed to lower cholesterol, and they may be beneficial as part of a healthy diet, but they would have to be eaten regularly to have a consistent, lasting effect.

LIFESTYLE

Lifestyle modifications, particularly diet and exercise, should be *the key* to your effort to reduce your cholesterol level. It's much healthier to address the problem with diet—which contributes to the problem in the first place—than it is to address it with medications that may not be necessary and carry the risk of side effects. Even if you do need medication, it should be prescribed in addition to—not in place of—diet and exercise. Research on the *reversal* of coronary atherosclerosis is based largely on diet, exercise, and stress reduction. This indicates that this trio of lifestyle changes may do more than simply lower cholesterol: it may have other significant health benefits.

Diet

Your cholesterol level is largely the result of what you eat. Cholesterol comes from two sources, both food sources. You either take it in directly from animal foods, or your liver manufactures it from the foods you eat, primarily fats. Although some people are genetically predisposed to high cholesterol levels, diet is generally one of the key factors in raising—and in lowering—cholesterol levels.

To reduce your cholesterol level with diet, all the major health organizations and experts agree that you need to limit your dietary cholesterol and fat, particularly saturated fat (the kind prevalent in animal foods like meat, eggs, and dairy products). The recommendations many people rely on produce only marginal improvements in cholesterol. For example, the U.S. government and many national health associations recommend a diet that gets 30 percent or less of its total calories from fat and restricts dietary cholesterol intake. The Step I diet, which these organizations generally recommend to start, limits dietary cholesterol to less than 300 milligrams per day and limits saturated fat intake to 8 to 10 percent of total calories. The Step II diet, which they recommend for further reduction or for people with extremely high cholesterol levels, limits dietary cholesterol to less than 200 milligrams per day and saturated fat intake to 7 percent or less of total calories. Although following these recommendations lowers cholesterol levels somewhat, this approach often proves inadequate. I believe—and research supports my position—that additional reductions in saturated fat and dietary cholesterol can result in additional important reductions in cholesterol levels. The reductions do not have to be painful. You don't have to give up all foods containing fat. You simply need to reorient your thinking—and your taste. For example, I used to drink whole milk. Now I drink skim milk. It took me a few weeks to get used to the different texture and taste, but now I can't stand the taste of whole milk. This type of reorientation occurs when you make simple substitutions to your diet. You don't have to "give up" everything. And you can eat quite a lot of food and keep your saturated fat intake low. I outline my dietary recommendations in detail in the next chapter.

In addition to reducing fat and cholesterol intake, you may want to consider adding certain foods to your diet. These foods can lower cholesterol levels. Soluble fiber, found in oat bran, oatmeal, apples, and beans, has been shown to help lower blood cholesterol levels in certain amounts. Soy, in particular, appears to have a beneficial effect. Some research indicates that an ounce of soy protein a day can reduce total cholesterol, LDL cholesterol, and triglycerides by 10 percent. It may also help raise HDL cholesterol. Garlic, too, has been shown in some studies to lower cholesterol levels, although other studies have found no such benefit. Still, it won't hurt to make liberal use of the herb in your cooking—as long as you have some mouthwash nearby.

Exercise

You already know that exercise is good for you, but you may not know that one of its many benefits is raising HDL cholesterol, the type that escorts LDL cholesterol out of the body. Exercise also helps you lose weight, which can also have a positive effect on your cholesterol levels, reducing LDL and triglycerides. If you have high blood cholesterol, you should consider a regular exercise program. It doesn't have to be intense. Even moderate physical activity can be beneficial if it's performed regularly (at least thirty minutes three or more days a week). I discuss some of the options available in the next chapter.

Stress Reduction

Although research on the subject is limited, excess stress has been shown to increase cholesterol levels. I believe stress probably plays a greater level in cholesterol levels—and the resulting atherosclerosis—than is recognized. Even if stress does not turn out to be a major player in cholesterol levels, you can't go wrong by taking steps to reduce stress. I discuss stress reduction in the "Stress" section later in this chapter and in chapter 5.

Clot in Heart

A number of heart conditions, including atrial fibrillation, valvular heart disease, and ventricular aneurysm, as well as certain blood disorders, can result in the development of a clot in the heart. This, obviously, is not good. It raises the risk of ischemic stroke above that caused by the underlying condition itself. If you have developed a clot in your heart, your doctor will probably recommend a two-pronged attack: one to treat the clot and one to eliminate its source. After all, you certainly don't want a new clot forming after you've taken care of the first. The treatment used to address the underlying condition depends on the condition itself. If atrial fibrillation is the cause, for example, treatment may include cardioversion to restore normal heart rhythm or anticoagulants to thin the blood and reduce the risk of clot formation. If valvular disease is the problem, the treatment could include surgery to repair or replace the valve, or anticoagulant therapy.

In the meantime, your doctor will want to address the clot that has formed. He or she can do that in one of two ways: surgically or medically.

Surgical

Depending on where the clot is located and the degree of risk it conveys, your doctor may recommend surgically removing it. Though this option, obviously, carries risks, it is one way to ensure that the clot is fully removed.

Medical

Another approach is to treat you with anticoagulants to thin the blood and prevent the formation of additional clots and monitor the existing clot with echocardiography to make sure it is not growing or moving.

Congenital Heart Defects

Congenital heart defects are heart defects that are present at birth. Sometimes they are the result of abnormal genes, sometimes of environmental factors during the child's development, and sometimes a combination of both. Some of these problems are detected before birth, some at birth, and some only when the person reaches adulthood, which demonstrates the varied nature of congenital heart defects. Some are serious and life-threatening; others have little or no effect on the heart's ability to function; and many fall in between. Heart defects can affect the blood vessels, the heart valves, the connections between the main arteries or veins and the heart, or the partitions between the heart's chambers. The number of defects is large, and each type of defect is treated differently. You need to discuss treatment for your particular defect with your cardiologist. The treatment may include surgery to repair a defect, surgery or medication to treat complications like congestive heart failure, and anticoagulants or antiplatelet agents to prevent clot development.

Congestive Heart Failure

Congestive heart failure is a condition in and of itself; it is often also the result of such other heart conditions as cardiomyopathy, ischemic heart disease, atrial fibrillation, hypertension, infection, and valvular heart disease. If the underlying cause is something that can be corrected—a diseased heart valve that can be repaired or replaced, an arrhythmia that can be corrected with cardioversion or a pacemaker, or a blocked coronary artery that can be opened with coronary artery bypass grafting or coronary angioplasty—treating that cause could reverse congestive heart failure. (I discuss the treatments for many of these conditions in other sections of this chapter.) In other cases, congestive heart failure is irreversible. In those instances, your doctor must focus on improving your heart's pumping ability, reducing its workload, and preventing clots, among other things, to reduce symptoms and to keep your heart functioning to the best of its ability. This is accomplished primarily with medications and lifestyle changes. When the heart becomes too weak to respond to conventional treatment, heart transplant becomes an option.

SURGICAL/INTERVENTIONAL

In addition to surgical or interventional procedures to treat the conditions that give rise to congestive heart failure, the other major surgical option for the condition is heart transplantation. Obviously, this is an extreme treatment. It is generally reserved for people in whom the heart is weakened to the point that it no longer responds to medication. Even with those restrictions, not all people will qualify. A limited number of donor hearts are available, so doctors take into consideration other factors, including your age, health, and willingness to comply with medical recommendations to determine if you are among those most likely to benefit from the procedure.

If you are recommended for a heart transplant, you will be placed on a waiting list for a heart to become available. When a healthy heart of a compatible blood type becomes available, you will be called to the hospital immediately to undergo the procedure. (The donated heart can remain outside the body for only four to six hours.) Once at the hospital, you will undergo tests to make sure that you are in a condition to handle surgery, then you will be given an anesthetic and connected to a heart-lung machine. The surgeon will remove your heart and replace it with the donor heart, connecting the new heart to your major arteries. The actual surgery is relatively straightforward, although, like any surgical procedure, it carries the risk of surgical complications, including reaction to the anesthetic and infection. In fact, the risk of infection is heightened, because you will have to take drugs to suppress your immune system to prevent it from rejecting the donated heart. You will have to take these medications and undergo regular screening for rejection for the rest of your life.

MEDICAL

Medications are the staples of treatment for congestive heart failure that cannot be corrected. Your doctor may recommend any of a number of medications, including positive inotropic medications to improve your heart's contraction strength, vasodilators to reduce the heart's workload, diuretics to reduce accumulated fluid, and anticoagulants to prevent blood clots.

Positive Inotropic Medications

These medications are designed to strengthen the heart's contraction strength. The most well-known of these medications is digitalis, which has been used to treat heart problems for more than two hundred years. Digitalis and related medications like digoxin (Lanoxin) increase the pumping strength of the heart and can help control certain rhythm disorders. Studies indicate that digitalis can help improve symptoms and reduce hospitalization for heart failure, although it has little or no effect on survival. Potential side effects include slow or irregular heartbeat, visual disturbances, loss of appetite, and stomach upset.

Vasodilators

Vasodilators are medications that dilate blood vessels. This enlarges them and reduces the amount of work the heart must do to pump blood through them. The primary vasodilators used to treat congestive heart failure are two classes of antihypertensive medications: such ACE inhibitors as captopril (Capoten), enlapril (Vasotec), and quinapril (Accupril), and such direct-acting vasodilators as hydralazine (Apresoline) and minoxidil (Loniten). I discuss the actions and side effects of these medications in detail in the "Hypertension" section on page 139. In terms of treating congestive heart failure, research has shown that vasodilators can effectively improve the heart's pumping efficiency and reduce symptoms. They can also prolong life. Since these drugs also lower blood pressure, you shouldn't take them if your blood pressure is already too low.

Diuretics

Congestive heart failure can cause fluid to accumulate in the legs, abdomen, liver, and lungs. This can cause shortness of breath and swelling. To ease these symptoms and help the body eliminate excess fluid, your doctor may prescribe diuretics. I describe these medications in detail in the "Hypertension" section. If your blood pressure is already too low, you should not take these medications.

Anticoagulants and Antiplatelet Agents

These medications thin the blood, making it flow more easily and reducing the likelihood of clot formation. This is important in congestive heart failure because the heart may be too weak to pump effectively, which can make blood flow sluggish. The most commonly prescribed anticoagulant for long-term use is warfarin (Coumadin). The primary side effect of this medication is bleeding or hemorrhage. If there is a strong contraindication to warfarin, such as hemorrhage, an antiplatelet medication may be used in its place.

LIFESTYLE

In addition to medications to treat congestive heart failure and treatments for underlying conditions, your doctor will likely tell you to take it easy and watch your sodium and fluid intake.

Activity

Although bed rest is no longer recommended as a permanent way of life for people with congestive heart failure, it has its role during episodes of severe symptoms. Today, most doctors will recommend that you remain some-what active to keep your body in shape, though you should not participate in activities that make you constantly short of breath.

Diet

You will likely be told to restrict your intake of both sodium and fluids. Sodium can reduce the effectiveness of certain medications. It can also promote fluid retention and high blood pressure. Fluids, too, must be restricted—the standard recommendation is no more than two quarts per day. This can help you combat the fluid retention that is common with heart failure.

Depression

Depression affects an estimated 15 million Americans each year. It not only affects their mood, it also affects their health. And it may increase their risk of ischemic stroke. Fortunately, depression can be overcome. Even without treatment, the majority of depressed people recover within six months to a year. Treatment—in the form of psychotherapy, pharmacotherapy (med-ications), or a combination—can shorten that recovery period significantly.

MEDICAL

Medications are available to prevent or relieve depression. These medica-tions, known as antidepressants, generally work by affecting brain chemicals that may be altered in people with depression. The various types of antide-pressants work somewhat differently, and one may work better than another for a particular person or a particular depressive condition. You and your doctor will have to work closely together to find which medication or medications are best for you if you determine that medication is the best way to treat your depression.

Tricyclic Antidepressants

These medications, also known as TCAs, are the oldest of the antidepres-sants. They work by raising levels of the brain chemicals serotonin and nor-epinephrine. They do this by slowing the rate at which nerve cells reabsorb the chemicals. It may take several weeks for TCAs, which include imip-ramine (Tofranil), amitriptyline (Elavil), and nortriptyline (Pamelor), to have their expected effect. Since TCAs have the potential to create cardio-vascular problems, people with a history of heart disease should avoid them. The medications can also pose problems for people who wear contact lenses (they decrease tear production), or who take thyroid supplements, certain antihypertensive medications, oral contraceptives, diuretics, antipsychotic drugs, and, in some cases, alcohol and tobacco. Potential side effects include dry mouth, constipation, urinary retention, weight gain, increased sweating, dizziness, fatigue, nausea, and heart palpitations, or arrhythmias.

Monoamine Oxidase Inhibitors

These medications work by blocking monoamine oxidase, an enzyme that destroys brain chemicals including norepinephrine and serotonin. These drugs, which include phenelzine (Nardil), tranylcypromine (Parnate), and isocarboxazid (Marplan), are often recommended for people who don't respond to tricyclic antidepressants and for people with atypical depression (a form characterized by overeating, oversleeping, lack of energy, and sensitivity to rejection). Potential side effects include dizziness, rapid heartbeat, and loss of sexual desire. In addition, these drugs can interact with certain foods, alcoholic beverages, and medications to produce a severe reaction that can increase blood pressure and lead to seizures, stroke, or coma. If your doctor prescribes an MAOI, make sure to get a list of the foods, beverages, and medications to avoid: it includes aged cheeses, processed meats, fish, and soy products, foods containing monosodium glutamate (MSG), red wines, some over-the-counter cold and allergy medications, local anesthetics, and insulin.

Selective Serotonin Reuptake Inhibitors

These medications, known as SSRIs, selectively block the reabsorption of the brain chemical serotonin. This class of antidepressants includes the popular drugs fluoxetine (Prozac), sertraline (Zoloft), and paroxetine (Paxil). These medications in general have fewer side effects than other types of antidepressants, although they can cause problems. Potential side effects include nausea, diarrhea, anxiety or nervousness, insomnia, headache, and rash.

Other Antidepressants

In addition to the three major classes of antidepressants, several others are also available. Venlafaxine (Effexor) and trazodone (Desyrel) are similar to SSRIs. Venlafaxine also blocks the reabsorption of norepinephrine. It has side effects similar to those of the TCAs and SSRIs. Trazodone is sedating, although it produces fewer side effects than the TCAs. A third drug, bupro-prion (Wellbutrin, Zyban), blocks the reabsorption of serotonin, dopa-mine, and norepinephrine. This drug is also used to help people quit smoking.

LIFESTYLE

The other primary treatment for depression is psychotherapy. Two primary types exist: insight-oriented therapy, which tries to help patients gain insight into the causes of their problems, and cognitive/behavioral therapy, which focuses on modifying behavior and thinking. These therapies do not have the potential for side effects that medications have. Their other advantage is that they can help you understand why you act and feel the way you do and help you gain control over behavior. Cognitive/behavioral therapy, for example, can include relaxation training, time management, and other techniques that can be helpful for managing stress. It may take longer to achieve results, and the treatment can be expensive. Psychotherapy is often used in conjunction with medication, which can reduce the length of treatment.

Diabetes Mellitus

This metabolic condition increases the risk of both ischemic stroke and ischemic heart disease. It is also a leading cause of kidney failure and blindness. Left untreated, diabetes can disable you, worsen your prognosis if you have a stroke, and shorten your life. Diabetes can be controlled. Doing so can significantly reduce your risk of ischemic stroke—as well as other diabetic complications. The burden of bringing the disease under control falls largely on you. Although you must work with a doctor to determine which treatments work best in your situation, day-to-day care for the disease is largely self-care.

Your treatment options for diabetes will depend largely on the type of diabetes you have. In type 1, or insulin-dependent diabetes, the body loses the ability to manufacture the hormone insulin. As a result, insulin replacement—usually in the form of injections—is a staple of treatment. In type 2, or non-insulin-dependent diabetes, the body produces insulin, but the hormone doesn't function properly. As a result, treatment may not require insulin; it may be accomplished with other medications or with lifestyle modifications. In fact, lifestyle changes play a major role in the control of both forms of diabetes.

MEDICAL

Medical treatment is required for type 1 diabetes and may be needed for type 2 diabetes, depending on its severity. The two types of medical treatments are the hormone insulin and medications known as oral hypoglycemic agents.

Insulin

This hormone enables the body to use glucose, a type of sugar, for energy. Without insulin, glucose builds up in the blood, and the body, starved for energy, begins to burn protein and fat. Both situations threaten health and, if left unchecked, can cause diabetic emergencies that may result in death. To prevent these emergencies and the long-term damage caused by high blood sugar, people with type 1 diabetes must take insulin on a regular basis. Some people with type 2 diabetes—notably those who cannot control their blood sugar level with other medications and diet and exercise—also must take insulin.

The hormone, which can be chemically produced, comes in three primary forms: short-acting (also called semilente or regular), which begins to work in thirty to forty-five minutes and lasts for five to eight hours; intermediate-acting (lente or NPH), which begins to work in about ninety minutes and lasts for eighteen to twenty-four hours; and long-acting (ultralente or PZI), which begins to work in four to twelve hours and lasts twenty to thirty-six hours. Many people use several forms of insulin, taken at different times throughout the day, to control their blood sugar. The hormone is usually administered by injection, though it can also be administered with a pump. The primary challenge in using insulin is to determine what type and dosage works best for you. You may be allergic to some types of insulin, or one type may work better than another. Time also plays a factor, as does your blood sugar level. You will have to monitor your blood sugar levels to determine when and how much insulin you need. You will also have to follow a diet and exercise plan. Insulin is not a medication you take in the morning and forget about until the next day. If you have type 1 diabetes or type 2 diabetes that cannot be controlled by other means, it's the mainstay of treatment.

Oral Hypoglycemic Agents

If you have type 2 diabetes, you may be able to control your condition with lifestyle modifications alone or a combination of lifestyle modifications and oral hypoglycemic agents. These are drugs that lower blood sugar levels. Although they are certainly more convenient than insulin, they do not work for everybody. They are most effective for people who develop diabetes after age forty and for people whose disease is newly discovered. Even when they have been effective, they may stop working after a period of time. Several types of these medications exist. Most are prescribed alone, but some can be prescribed in combination.

The sulfonylureas, which include acetohexamide (Dymelor), chlorpropamide (Diabinese), glimepiride (Amaryl), glipizide (Glucotrol), glyburide (DiaBeta, Glynase), tolazamide, and tolbutamide, stimulate the pancreas to produce more insulin, which in turn lowers blood sugar levels. If you take one of these medications, you must monitor your blood sugar level to make sure it doesn't fall too low. The drugs may also promote weight gain.

The biguanide family, which includes metformin, works by causing the liver to reduce stored glucose more slowly. Side effects of this medication include nausea, diarrhea, and loss of appetite. In people with heart, kidney, or liver disease, it can also cause a life-threatening buildup of acid in the blood. Biguanides do not promote weight gain and only occasionally cause blood sugar levels to drop to dangerous levels.

Alpha-glucosidase inhibitors, a new family of drugs, slow the digestion of food, which in turn slows glucose's entry into the bloodstream. The best-known drug in this class is acarbose. Side effects of acarbose include gas, abdominal pain, and diarrhea. The drug does not promote weight gain or produce hypoglycemia (low blood sugar).

Another new family of drugs, the meglitinide class, stimulates the production of insulin. The first drug in this class, repaglinide, is generally taken before a meal. Its side effects, like those of the sulfonylureas, include weight gain and hypoglycemia. It can be used in combination with other hypoglycemic drugs.

Rosiglitazone (Avandia), another relatively new drug, increases the body's sensitivity to insulin. Its side effects include headache, abdominal pain, and liver abnormalities, and it can be used alone or in combination with other drugs.

LIFESTYLE

Lifestyle modifications—most notably diet and exercise—are crucial if you have diabetes. They may constitute your sole method of control, or they may be part of an overall treatment program that includes insulin or oral hypoglycemic agents.

Diet

Diabetes affects how the body uses food, so it should come as no surprise that what you eat—and when—plays a role in controlling the disease. If you have diabetes, you need to work with your doctor or a nutrition expert or a dietician to determine what changes you need to make in your diet. You will likely be advised to eat a diet that is low in fat and cholesterol, moderate in protein, and high in fiber. You will probably be asked to pay attention to the carbohydrates you eat—particularly simple carbohydrates that can cause a quick rise in your blood sugar level. This doesn't mean that you can't eat sugar, as many people think. It simply means that you have to be aware that sugar or foods that contain sugar rapidly increase blood sugar levels and take that into consideration when you choose what and when to eat. What and when you eat are extremely important in diabetes: they play a role in the timing and dose of insulin and other medications and vice versa. You can see why I said lifestyle modifications are crucial and why I said that much of the responsibility for controlling diabetes falls on you. You will need to work with your doctor to determine the best combination of lifestyle and medical treatments.

Exercise

Exercise also plays a role in controlling diabetes: it lowers blood sugar. It also has numerous other benefits, including speeding weight loss, improving cardiovascular health, building muscle tone, and reducing stress. It is generally recommended as a part of a comprehensive treatment program for diabetes—in fact, it may help some people with type 2 diabetes avoid being treated with medication or insulin. It also may reduce insulin needs in people who take it. Since exercise lowers blood sugar, you should check with your doctor before launching into an exercise program. If you take insulin, you will need to determine how your food intake and insulin dose should be adjusted as a result of exercise. You may also need to carry a high-sugar snack to combat hypoglycemia if exercise reduces your blood sugar excessively. You should also know when not to exercise, such as when your blood sugar level is more than 300 mg/dL, when your medication is reaching its peak effectiveness, and when you are ill or injured.

Diet

A poor diet can contribute to several major stroke risk factors, including hypertension, atherosclerosis, and diabetes. Fortunately, a good diet—notably one that is low in sodium, cholesterol, and saturated fat and high in fruits and vegetables—can help prevent stroke. I explain my recommendations for a brain-healthy diet in detail in the next chapter.

Disorders That Cause Increased Clotting

Blood diseases that thicken the blood or make it more likely to clot increase the risk of ischemic stroke. These conditions, though not widespread, are numerous. They include polycythemia, thrombocythemia, thrombocytopenic purpura, dysproteinemia, antiphospholipid antibody syndrome, leukemia, and disseminated intravascular coagulation. The treatment for each of these conditions obviously varies. I describe some of the interventional and medical treatments that are used to treat these conditions and give you several examples of what you may expect, but you will have to work with your doctor to determine the type of treatment most appropriate for your own condition.

SURGICAL/INTERVENTIONAL

Although surgery is not commonly performed to treat blood disorders, it is possible. Some cases of thrombotic thrombocytopenic purpura, for example, may be treated by removing the spleen, a procedure known as *splenec-*

tomy. Most blood disorders are more likely to be treated with one of several interventional procedures to reduce the blood's tendency to clot: phlebotomy, apheresis, and infusion.

Phlebotomy

Phlebotomy may sound like a complex medical procedure, but it is simply the removal of blood from a vein. You've experienced this procedure if you've ever had a blood test or donated blood. It involves inserting a needle into a vein and withdrawing blood. Generally, it is performed to obtain blood for some diagnostic purpose. In the case of certain blood diseases, however, it is a treatment in itself. Phlebotomy reduces the amount of circulating blood. It is the primary treatment for polycythemia, an elevated level of red blood cells. It is also the first step in apheresis.

Apheresis

Apheresis is a procedure in which blood is temporarily removed, and one or more components are removed from it before it is reinfused back into the patient. In *plasmapheresis,* plasma is removed. This procedure is sometimes used to treat thrombocytopenic purpura (low number of platelets), dysproteinemia (abnormal protein content), and, on rare occasions, antiphospholipid antibody syndrome (antibodies that affect clotting). In *plateletpheresis,* platelets are removed. This may be used to treat thrombocythemia (elevated platelet count).

Infusion

In this procedure, blood or certain blood components are given to a patient. This is the final step of apheresis, but it is also a treatment in and of itself. If you have thrombocytopenic purpura, for example, you may be given an infusion of fresh frozen plasma (which contains platelets) to help you compensate for the decreased number of platelets in your blood.

MEDICATIONS

As you might expect, medications such as anticoagulants and antiplatelet agents can play a role in treating certain blood conditions. These drugs thin the blood and reduce the risk of clotting. They are often used to treat antiphospholipid antibody syndromes, in which antibodies in the blood affect clotting. (Since these syndromes also involve inflammation, corticosteroids may also be used to treat them.) The most commonly prescribed anticoagulant is warfarin (Coumadin). Its primary side effect is a tendency to cause bleeding or hemorrhage. Antiplatelet agents like aspirin and clopidogrel, which thin the blood in a different and less effective way, are less likely to cause bleeding.

Endocarditis

Endocarditis is an inflammation of the endocardium, the membrane that lines the heart and valves. Usually caused by a bacterial infection of a heart valve, it can lead to the development of blood clots that can make their way to the brain and cause ischemic stroke. It is also associated with the development of mycotic intracranial aneurysms, which increase the risk of subarachnoid hemorrhage. Those most likely to develop endocarditis are those with valvular heart diseases, like mitral valve disease, those with congenital heart defects that affect the valves, and those who have an artificial heart valve. These people are at increased risk of developing an infection. Bacteria that may enter their bloodstream from a dental or surgical procedure, or even a minor gum injury, can migrate to the heart and cause a problem. This is why these people are often cautioned to take prophylactic antibiotics before undergoing surgical or dental procedures.

Antibiotics are the mainstay of treatment for endocarditis. The choice of drug depends on the type of bacteria that are causing the infection. Some bacteria are resistant to certain types of antibiotics.

Exercise

Inactivity is a risk factor for all types of ischemic stroke. This risk can be easily reduced with regular exercise. I discuss my exercise prescription in the next chapter.

Hypertension

Hypertension is a strong risk factor for ischemic and hemorrhagic stroke. It is also one of the most common stroke risk factors. More than 50 million Americans have hypertension, though approximately one-third of them don't know it. Fortunately, reducing blood pressure has been shown conclusively to reduce stroke risk. In fact, the decline in stroke incidence and mortality that we had been experiencing through the mid-1990s is attributed, at least in part, to increased control of hypertension. That decline has plateaued. In the past ten years or so, we have actually seen a decline in the awareness of treatment and control of hypertension. This trend is alarming not only because hypertension—which may be a reflection of endothelial dysfunction—can have serious consequences, but also because it can be controlled. This is generally accomplished by lifestyle modifications and, if necessary, medications.

MEDICAL

Although control of high blood pressure should start with lifestyle modifications, numerous medications are available if changes fail to bring blood pressure to the desired level. This does not mean that medication should replace lifestyle changes: the two should go hand in hand. Although lifestyle modifications are not always able to eliminate the need for medication, they can often reduce that need. I firmly believe that it's better to reduce our reliance on medications whenever possible. We should never forget the important role our lifestyle plays on our health—for better or worse. That said, medications have an important role in the control of blood pressure— and in preventing stroke. Numerous types of medications are available, and the numbers are constantly growing. The choice of medication is important and should be made based upon your own individual situation; these drugs can have other effects, both positive and negative, on your health. Ideally, blood pressure should be controlled with a single daily dose of one antihypertensive medication. Additional doses or medications may be added if one medication is unable to reduce pressure to the desired levels.

ACE Inhibitors

These drugs have multiple effects on the cardiovascular system. Officially known as angiotensin converting enzyme inhibitors, they interfere with the production of angiotensin, a chemical that causes arteries to constrict. This strengthens the heart's pumping action and reduces blood pressure. They are the preferred blood pressure treatment for people who also have congestive heart failure. In fact, they are also used to treat heart failure. They are also recommended as a first-line treatment for people who have diabetes with proteinuria (large amounts of protein in the urine). They are not recommended for people with certain vascular kidney problems, including a narrowing, or stenosis, of the renal artery, or for women who are pregnant. And they are generally less effective in African Americans.

ACE inhibitors include captopril (Capoten), moexipril (Univasc), enalpril (Vasotec), lisinopril (Zestril, Prinivil), quinapril (Accupril), benazepril (Lotensin), fosinopril (Monopril), ramipril (Altace), and trandolapril (Mavik). These medications can produce side effects, including a persistent, dry cough; rash; loss of taste; angioedema, or swelling; high potassium levels; and stomach upset.

Alpha Agonists

These medications, also known as alpha 2 agonists and centrally acting alpha 2 agonists, block nerve receptors that promote the constriction of small blood vessels. This causes the vessels to dilate, which lowers blood pressure. These drugs include methyldopa (Aldomet), guanfacine (Tenex), and clonidine (Catapres). They are recommended as first-line antihypertensive treatment in people with high cholesterol and in men with benign prostatic hypertrophy, or enlarged prostate. Possible side effects include dizziness, insomnia, nausea, fluid retention, dry mouth, rash, and liver function abnormalities.

Angiotensin II Inhibitors

This new class of drugs blocks angiotensin II, the product of angiotensin and angiotensin converting enzyme and, possibly, other enzymes. This chemical has been found to harm the heart and kidney and increase the risk of stroke and heart attack. Angiotensin II inhibitors, also known as ACE II inhibitors, block the actions of this chemical, lowering blood pressure as a result. They may also reduce heart enlargement and have a favorable effect on heart failure. Six of these medications have been approved by the Food and Drug Administration: losartan (Cozaar, Hyzaar), valsartan (Diovan, Tareg, Nisis), irbesartan (Aprovel, Avapro, Karvea), candesartan (Atacand, Kenzen, Blopress), telmisartan (Micardis, Pritor), and eprosartan (Teveten).

The blood pressure–lowering benefits of angiotensin II inhibitors are similar to those of ACE inhibitors, and there are fewer side effects; dry cough, the most common side effect of ACE inhibitors, is not a problem with angiotensin II inhibitors. Since these drugs are relatively new and their long-term effects are unknown, the Joint National Committee on Detection, Evaluation and Treatment of High Blood Pressure, a panel convened by the National Heart, Lung and Blood Institute, recommends that they be used primarily for people who should take ACE inhibitors but cannot tolerate them for some reason.

Beta-Blockers

These drugs, along with diuretics, are recommended as first-line hypertension treatment for people without additional conditions. They slow the heartbeat and reduce the contraction strength of the heart, which reduces the heart's need for oxygen; they also lower blood pressure and, in some cases, restore irregular heart rhythm to normal. These workhorses of cardiovascular medicine are used to treat heart attack, angina, and certain rhythm disorders as well as to lower blood pressure. As a result, they are the preferred hypertension treatment for anyone who also has had a heart attack or been diagnosed with angina or atrial fibrillation. They also have benefits for people who suffer from migraines and people with an overactive thyroid. They are not recommended for people who have depression, diabetes, low heart rate, heart block, sick sinus syndrome, high cholesterol, asthma, chronic obstructive pulmonary disease, or peripheral vascular disease (intermittent claudication). They should be used with caution in people with congestive heart failure and are generally less effective in African Americans.

Beta-blockers include propranolol (Inderal), metoprolol (Lopressor), nadolol (Corgard), atenolol (Tenormin), acebutolol (Sectral), betaxolol (Kerlone), labetalol (Normodyne, Trandate), penbutolol (Levatol), pindolol (Visken), timolol (Blocadren), cartelolol (Cartrol), bisoprolol (Zebeta), and sotalol (Betapace). Their possible side effects include an abnormally slow heart rate, bronchospasm, depression, fatigue, weakness, dizziness, insomnia, indigestion, and decreased libido. In addition, you should not abruptly stop taking these drugs; abrupt withdrawal could predispose you to heart attack.

Calcium Channel Blockers

Calcium channel blockers block the passage of calcium into the heart and blood vessels, which ultimately affects the size of the blood vessels. Calcium channel blockers have multiple effects on the heart: they reduce heart rate and lower the heart's contraction strength, which reduces the heart's need of oxygen; they dilate the coronary arteries, which increases oxygen flow to the heart; and, in some cases, they restore irregular heart rhythm to normal. Of course, they also reduce blood pressure. Calcium channel blockers are often recommended as first-line antihypertensive treatment for people with angina and atrial fibrillation. They are also particularly beneficial for people with isolated systolic hypertension (an increase in the upper number of the blood pressure reading), people with diabetes and proteinurea (high levels of protein in the urine), and people with migraine headaches. And they may be more effective than ACE inhibitors and beta-blockers for African Americans.

These drugs, which include verapamil (Calan, Isoptin, Verelan), nifedipine (Procardia, Adalat), nicardipine (Cardene), diltiazem (Cardizem, Dilacor), isradipine (DynaCirc), mibefradil (Posicor), felodipine (Plendil), bepridil (Vascor), amlodipine (Norvasc), and nisoldipine (Sular), can cause excessively slow heartbeat, constipation, headache, swelling in the legs, and flushing.

Direct Vasodilators

As their name implies, these medications directly cause the blood vessels to relax and dilate. This reduces the heart's workload and decreases blood pressure. These drugs, which include hyrdalazine (Apresoline) and minoxidil (Loniten), are generally taken in conjunction with diuretics and beta-blockers because they cause fluid retention and rapid heart rate. Other possible side effects include headache, diarrhea, flushing, symptoms that resemble lupus, and, in the case of minoxidil, hair growth on the face and body. (Incidentally, this side effect is what led to the use of minoxidil as a treatment for hair loss.)

Diuretics

Diuretics are among the earliest antihypertensive medications used. These medications speed up the elimination of fluids from the body, which reduces blood pressure and swelling. Like beta-blockers, diuretics are recommended as first-line treatment for people with hypertension and no additional conditions. Because they increase the effectiveness of other antihypertensive medications, they are also generally the first choice for a second drug, if a second drug is needed. Diuretics, which are also used to treat congestive heart failure, are a good choice for people who have heart failure in addition to hypertension. They are also of particular benefit for people with isolated systolic hypertension. They are often a good first-line choice for African Americans because they are generally more effective, than ACE inhibitors and beta-blockers in this setting. Low-dose diuretics also have benefits for people with type 2 diabetes, but diuretics are not recommended for people with gout or kidney insufficiency.

Many diuretics are on the market. Some deplete the body of potassium; others, known as potassium-sparing diuretics, have less effect on potassium levels. Some of the diuretics used to treat hypertension include chlorthalidone (Hygroton, Thaliton), chlorothiazide (Diuril), hydrochlorothiazide (Esidrix), methylchlothiazide (Aquatensin, Enduron), and metalazone (Diulo, Zaroxolyn). These medications may result in low potassium and sodium levels and high levels of calcium and blood sugar, as well as stomach upset and gout. Potassium-sparing diuretics, including amiloride (Midamor), spironolactone (Aldactone), triamterene (Dyrenium, Diazide), bendroflumethiazide, benzthiazide, indapamide, quinethazone, polythiazide, trichlormethiazide, and hydroflumethiazide, can decrease or, rarely, increase potassium levels. They also can cause stomach upset. A third category of diuretics, called loop diuretics, are used to treat hypertension related to kidney disease. These drugs, which include bumatanide (Bumex), ethacrynic acid (Edecrin), furosemide (Lasix), and torsemide (Demadex), quickly reduce excess fluid. In fact, their side effects include excess fluid output and low blood pressure, as well as low potassium, calcium, and sodium, high blood sugar, gout, stomach upset, and muscle cramps.

Peripheral Adrenergic Agonists

These medications block the release or effect of adrenaline, a stimulating hormone the body releases in response to stress. Excess adrenaline increases blood pressure, while reduced amounts lower it. These drugs, which include guanadrel (Hylorel), guanethidine (Ismelin), mecamylamine (Inversine), prazosin (Minipress), rauwolfia alkaloids (Harmonyl, Raudixin, Rauzid, Serpasil), terazosin (Hytril), and doxazosin (Cardura), can significantly reduce blood pressure, especially after exercise. You may need to stand slowly to avoid a sudden drop in blood pressure if you are taking one of these medications. They can also cause fluid retention, dizziness, drowsiness, depression, and stomach upset.

LIFESTYLE

Lifestyle modifications are a staple of hypertension treatment, even if medication is required. Diet and exercise have the potential to prevent hypertension from occurring in the first place. If you already have hypertension, they, along with smoking cessation and a reduction in body weight, may be able to lower your blood pressure so that you do not need medication. Even if they are not effective alone, they can reduce the number and/or dose of the medications you must take. And they have other positive effects on the body—including independently reducing your risk of atherosclerosis and ischemic stroke.

Diet

Obesity is a risk factor for hypertension, and diet clearly has an effect on body weight. A diet high in calories, fat, and cholesterol promotes weight gain. A diet high in fat and cholesterol also promotes atherosclerosis, which is often seen along with hypertension. The two conditions increase the risk of ischemic heart disease and ischemic stroke. Even if you are not overweight and don't have atherosclerosis, it makes sense to reduce your fat and cholesterol intake. It's simply a matter of doing what's right for your body.

Additional dietary factors also come into play when it comes to hypertension. Sodium, one of the two main components of salt, for example, causes blood pressure to rise in sodium-sensitive individuals. The typical American diet contains far too much sodium. Cutting back on your sodium intake may help you reduce your blood pressure. On the flip side, make sure to get enough potassium, calcium, and magnesium. These minerals may help you keep blood pressure under control. And, as I explain above, some antihypertensive medications, like diuretics, deplete the body's supply of potassium. Research indicates that increasing your consumption of fruits and vegetables may also help keep blood pressure in control. Finally, you may want to reduce your intake of caffeine. Caffeine is known to cause rapid, temporary rises in high blood pressure. Though caffeine has not been found to cause chronic hypertension, if your blood pressure level is already high, you may not want it to rise any more, even if the jump is only temporarily. I discuss my recommendations for a diet to prevent stroke in detail in the next chapter. These recommendations can also help you prevent or control hypertension.

Alcohol

Alcohol, too, can have an effect on blood pressure. In large doses, it causes blood pressure to rise. Excessive intake can also alter the effectiveness of antihypertensive medications. However, alcohol may have a protective effect on the heart and blood vessels, reducing the risk of heart attack and atherosclerotic ischemic stroke. Since atherosclerosis and hypertension often go hand in hand, I don't want to discourage you from having an occasional drink to reap the potential benefits of alcohol, but I do want to caution you not to overdo it. Limit your intake to two drinks or fewer per day.

Exercise

Exercise is another potent tool in the prevention and control of hypertension. Quite simply, exercise helps lower blood pressure. It may do this independently or by causing weight loss. It also helps reduce stress, which can cause blood pressure to rise. And it strengthens your heart. This is just the tip of the iceberg. Exercise can also give you a mental boost, increase your energy level, and reduce fatigue, among other things. The most beneficial type of exercise for hypertension is aerobic exercise, the kind that requires oxygen and improves cardiovascular health. You should strive for thirty to forty-five minutes of such aerobic activity as walking, running, swimming, or dancing three to five times a week. Isometric exercise, including some forms of weight lifting, is less beneficial for cardiovascular health and, in some cases, may be harmful because it causes a sharp, temporary increase in blood pressure. I discuss exercise in more detail in the next chapter.

Weight Reduction

Being overweight is a risk factor for hypertension. If you are overweight, you should consider losing weight. Depending on how heavy you are, losing as little as ten pounds can reduce your blood pressure. Weight loss also enhances the effectiveness of blood pressure medications, and it makes you feel better about yourself. Following the dietary changes and exercise recommendations in chapter 5 can help you lose weight and keep it off.

Hypokinetic/Akinetic Heart Segment

Hypokinetic/akinetic heart segment is an impaired movement of the heart's left ventricle (lower chamber) that usually occurs as the result of a heart attack. This impaired area of the heart may lead to the formation of a clot in the heart, which, in turn, could lead to cardioembolic ischemic stroke. Periodic clinical follow-up for the development of a clot is often undertaken (treatment for an actual clot is described in the "Clot in the Heart" section on page 127), and treatment with such antiplatelet agents as aspirin or clopidogrel (Plavix) to prevent clots from developing (see "Antiplatelet Agents" on page 104). These medications thin the blood. Because of that action, they carry a minor risk of causing intracerebral hemorrhage.

If hypokinetic/akinetic heart segment occurs in conjunction with congestive heart failure, treatment could also include such positive inotropic agents as digitalis and digoxin (Lanoxin). These medications, described in detail in the "Congestive Heart Failure" section on page 128, are designed to improve the heart's contraction strength.

Intermittent Claudication

Intermittent claudication is a predictable, recurring pain in the leg. The pain occurs because the muscles in the leg aren't getting enough oxygen and nutrients. This deprivation is usually caused by atherosclerosis, which, as you know, is a risk factor for ischemic stroke. The focus of treatment for intermittent claudication itself is reducing the pain and preventing atherosclerosis from progressing in the leg. (In severe cases, the disease can block one of the leg arteries, causing gangrene and requiring amputation.) These treatments include medications such as cilostazol (Pletal) and pentoxifylline (Trental), designed to increase the distance a person can walk before experiencing symptoms, and angioplasty to clear a blockage in a leg. They also include lifestyle modifications to slow or stop the progression of atherosclerosis in general. These are the treatments that can help reduce your risk of ischemic stroke.

LIFESTYLE

The two primary therapies for intermittent claudication are exercise and smoking cessation. In addition, you should consider eating a very low-fat, low-cholesterol diet to slow the progression of atherosclerosis. Your doctor may also test and treat you for other conditions that could have an effect on intermittent claudication, such as diabetes and high cholesterol. If you have diabetes mellitus, your doctor will work with you to bring your blood sugar levels under control. And if you have high cholesterol, your doctor will recommend a diet and, perhaps, medications, to reduce these levels. I discuss controlling blood sugar and cholesterol levels, respectively, in the sections "Diabetes Mellitus" and "Cholesterol and Triglyceride Levels."

Exercise

Exercise may be very beneficial for individuals with intermittent claudication. Regular exercise conditions your muscles, which reduces the amount of oxygen they require. It also improves blood flow to the smaller arteries in the leg. Depending on the severity of your condition, you may be able to start your own exercise program—walking, climbing stairs, or riding a stationary bike for about thirty minutes three or more times a week. Stop at the point when you feel pain. If pain occurs within a very brief time, you may benefit from a more formal, supervised exercise program in which you walk on a treadmill for several minutes until pain begins, stop, rest, then go back to the treadmill. You repeat the cycle of exercise and rest until you've accumulated thirty to sixty minutes of walking. And you do this three times a week. Research indicates that up to 70 percent of people who start a regular exercise program can walk farther within six months to a year.

Smoking Cessation

If you have intermittent claudication and you smoke, consider quitting. You can reduce your risk of having a leg amputated tenfold. See "Smoking" for suggestions on how to quit. You should also avoid passive smoke.

Diet

A diet high in fat and cholesterol leads to the development of atherosclerotic plaque in the arteries. If you have intermittent claudication, you probably already have a buildup. To stop this buildup from progressing—and perhaps reverse it—you should eat a diet that is low in both fat and cholesterol. Research among people with atherosclerosis of the coronary arteries indicates that atherosclerosis can be stopped or reversed with a diet that restricts fat intake to less than 10 percent of total calories and cholesterol intake to less than 5 milligrams per day. Although studies have not yet indicated whether such a diet can reverse atherosclerotic buildup in other arteries, including those in the legs, I believe it makes sense to reduce fat and cholesterol intake to levels somewhat comparable to those. I discuss dietary recommendations in detail in the next chapter.

Intracranial Aneurysm

If you have an unruptured intracranial aneurysm, you are at increased risk of subarachnoid hemorrhage and, to a lesser extent, intracerebral hemorrhage. Rupture of an intracranial aneurysm is the leading cause of subarachnoid hemorrhage. Unruptured aneurysms have the potential to rupture. Although this can be frightening, it does not mean that you are a walking time bomb. After all, most intracranial aneurysms never rupture. In fact, the International Study of Unruptured Intracranial Aneurysms has found that unruptured aneurysms generally have a more benign prognosis than was previously thought. Specifically, the study found that people with small unruptured aneurysms (less than 10 millimeters or approximately ⅖ of an inch) and no history of other ruptured aneurysms have a risk of rupture of only ½₀ of 1 percent per year. This is clearly good news. In general, it means that people in this situation can lead a normal lifestyle with minimal risk while monitoring their aneurysm. Certain factors, including warning leaks, the presence of other symptoms, and the size and location of the aneurysm, can increase the risk of rupture. I encourage you to talk with your doctor about your condition. Together, you can determine whether you would benefit from a surgical procedure to repair the aneurysm or whether you would be better off undergoing regular monitoring and making modest lifestyle changes to reduce the risk of rupture.

SURGICAL AND INTERVENTIONAL

The traditional method of repairing an intracranial aneurysm is surgical clipping. In recent years, several high-tech endovascular procedures also have become available. Any of these procedures can be lifesaving for people whose aneurysms are in imminent danger of rupture. However, they are difficult procedures, and they do carry significant risk. You and your doctor will have to compare your risk of rupture to the risks posed by these procedures to determine if any are right for you.

Clipping

This traditional repair method, which involves clipping the neck of the aneurysm to isolate it from the artery's circulation, is still the procedure most commonly used to repair an aneurysm and prevent it from rupturing. It can prevent hemorrhagic stroke, particularly in younger people with large aneurysms who are experiencing aneurysm symptoms other than rupture. However, it is not without risk. Surgical clipping is a form of brain surgery. In addition to traditional surgical risks, such as infection and reaction to anesthesia, it carries risks such as aneurysm rupture, hemorrhage, and lasting neurological deficits. Death is also a possibility. It must be performed by a skilled surgeon, and the risks and benefits must clearly be weighed.

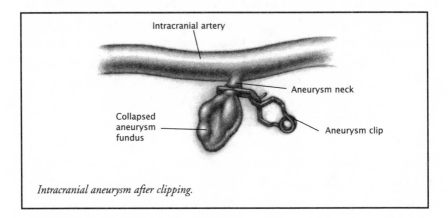

Intracranial aneurysm after clipping.

The procedure is most beneficial in people for whom the risk of rupture is high. This includes people who have experienced symptoms other than rupture (described in chapter 3), people whose aneurysms are large, and people who have a history of rupture from a different aneurysm. Unruptured aneurysms more than 25 millimeters in diameter are particularly prone to rupture. The International Study of Unruptured Intracranial Aneurysms reported in December 1998 that among patients with no history of rupture from a separate aneurysm, rupture rates correlate with the size of the aneurysm as follows:

- aneurysms 25 millimeters or greater: 1 to 2 percent per year (6 percent in the first year)
- aneurysms between 10 and 24 millimeters: a little less than 1 percent per year
- aneurysms smaller than 10 millimeters: $\frac{1}{20}$ of 1 percent per year

Particularly for people with smaller aneurysms, the risk of surgery may be considerably higher than the risk of rupture. The study found that the overall risk of death or serious neurological complications from surgery to repair an aneurysm is about 15.7 percent at one year for people with no history of rupture and about 13.2 percent at one year after surgery for people with a history of rupture. If you have had a subarachnoid hemorrhage from another intracranial aneurysm, the procedure is more likely to be beneficial even for a small aneurysm, particularly if you are younger (less than forty-five years old). The study found that the risk of rupture increases to $\frac{1}{2}$ of 1 percent per year in people with small aneurysms and a history of rupture.

Age also should play a role in determining whether to operate. The risks of the procedure increase with increasing age. The International Study of Unruptured Intracranial Aneurysms recently found that the one-year risk of major complications from surgery is 6.5 percent in people under age forty-five, 14.4 percent in people ages forty-five to sixty-four, and 32 percent in people sixty-five and older. As with any major surgical procedure, overall health should also be considered.

Endovascular Procedures

Endovascular procedures can also be used to repair aneurysms and may be an option. Although these high-tech procedures are not as widely available as open surgery, they are becoming increasingly popular. They are particularly useful when surgical clipping is not feasible, for instance, when an aneurysm is located in a hard-to-access area. These procedures, which include inserting metallic coils through a catheter into an aneurysm so a clot can form in the aneurysm and isolate it from the circulation and, less commonly, inserting a balloon in the parent artery above or below the aneurysm to isolate it, do carry risks. In some cases, endovascular procedures may be advantageous over and above surgical clipping, but this needs to be better studied to determine in which circumstances this is the case.

MEDICAL

Conservative management of intracranial aneurysms involves regular monitoring with imaging scans and efforts to prevent rupture. Although no medications are available to treat unruptured aneurysms or to prevent them from rupturing, medications that sharply increase blood pressure may, at least theoretically, increase the risk of aneurysm rupture. If you have an unruptured aneurysm, you should talk with your doctor or pharmacist about any medications you are taking—prescription or nonprescription. If any are known to cause rapid increases in blood pressure, a substitution may be in order. If you suffer from allergies, for example, you may be able to take an antihistamine like diphenhydramine (Benadryl) rather than a decongestant like pseudoephedrine. You should also talk with your doctor about any anticoagulants or antiplatelet agents you may be taking. Although it is not clear that these blood-thinning medications will cause an aneurysm to rupture, they could make the bleeding from a rupture worse. If you have an unruptured aneurysm, take acetaminophen (Tylenol) instead of aspirin when you need an over-the-counter pain reliever or fever reducer.

LIFESTYLE

If you are not a candidate for surgery, you can make lifestyle changes that reduce your risk of rapidly increasing your blood pressure and, thus, reduce your risk of aneurysm rupture. Even if you are a candidate for surgery, you should consider one lifestyle change—smoking cessation.

Smoking Cessation

Although smoking has not been conclusively linked to future rupture of unruptured aneurysms, the possibility exists. Even more important is that smoking has been linked to the development of unruptured intracranial aneurysms. Since intracranial aneurysms are most prone to rupture shortly after they form, smoking cessation could reduce your risk of developing a

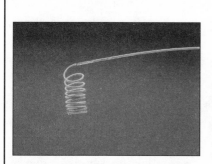

A. A tiny metal coil is used to isolate an intracranial aneurysm from the blood supply.

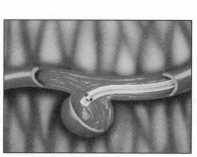

B. A catheter, or hollow tube, is inserted through the artery to the aneurysm.

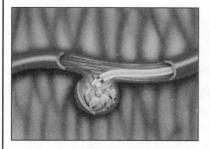

C. The metal coil is inserted through the catheter into the aneurysm, where it begins to open.

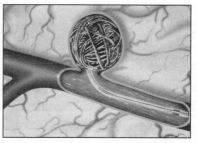

D. The coil continues to spring open, filling the aneurysm.

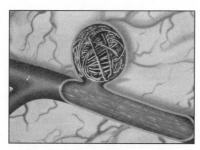

E. After the catheter is removed, the coil remains and allows clot to form in the aneurysm to isolate it from the circulation.

A coiling procedure is also used to treat intracranial aneurysms.

new aneurysm, which could reduce your risk of hemorrhagic stroke. I discuss various methods to help you quit on page 169. You should also try to avoid passive smoke.

Stress Reduction

Stress is known to spike blood pressure, and there is some evidence that temporary, rapid increases in blood pressure may cause an aneurysm to rupture. For these reasons, if you have an unruptured aneurysm, it's wise to pay attention to your stress level and take steps to reduce it. Stress reduction has other benefits as well. I discuss stress reduction in detail in chapter 5.

Straining Avoidance

As I've said, rapid spikes in blood pressure may increase the risk of aneurysm rupture. Although usual day-to-day exercise and activities, including sexual activity, do not appear to be a problem, activities that cause you to strain can produce these spikes. If you have an unruptured aneurysm, you should think twice before performing such activities. Don't try to install the heavy room air conditioner single-handedly, for example. Use a stool softener if constipation causes you to strain. And consider aerobic exercise rather than isometric exercise. Mild amounts of strength training with weights are probably not a problem, but don't strive to win a Charles Atlas contest.

Caffeine Avoidance

Although we're more likely to think of caffeine as a food additive, it is also a drug. We find this drug in our coffee, our soft drinks, our chocolate, our pain relievers. Regardless of whether we ingest caffeine for pleasure or as an ingredient of over-the-counter medication, it causes a temporary increase in blood pressure and, thus, has the potential to increase the risk of aneurysm rupture. Cutting back your caffeine intake to two cups or less of a caffeinated beverage—or avoiding it altogether—could reduce your risk of hemorrhagic stroke.

Alcohol Avoidance

Alcohol consumption, particularly heavy alcohol consumption and binge drinking, has been linked to both types of hemorrhagic stroke. If you drink heavily or binge drink, you should consider reducing your alcohol intake or avoiding alcohol altogether. I discuss ways to reduce alcohol consumption on page 97.

Ischemic Heart Disease

Ischemic heart disease, also known as coronary artery disease, is generally caused by atherosclerotic buildup in the coronary arteries. This buildup blocks or reduces the flow of blood and oxygen to the heart, resulting in the chest pain known as angina or, in more severe cases, heart attack. Heart attack, as I've explained, can result in the development of a blood clot that travels to the arteries in the brain, causing ischemic stroke. Ischemic heart disease also indicates the presence of atherosclerosis, which, as you know, can also cause ischemic stroke. If you've been diagnosed with ischemic heart disease, coronary artery disease, or coronary artery blockage, you need to take steps to prevent heart attack and steps to slow the progression of atherosclerosis. Doing so can not only reduce your risk of ischemic stroke but also reduce your risk of dying from heart disease.

Treatments for ischemic heart disease abound, from surgery to medication to adopting a heart-healthy lifestyle. I provide a brief description of the options here, but if you have ischemic heart disease, you need to work closely with a cardiologist to determine the approach that works best for you. The condition should be treated for its own sake—not simply to reduce your risk of ischemic stroke.

Surgical/Interventional

The surgical and interventional procedures used to treat ischemic heart disease are generally reserved for people whose symptoms are not relieved by medications and lifestyle changes and for people who are at high risk for heart attack or death; this includes people with blockages of the left main coronary artery and people with blockages of all three coronary arteries. The two interventional procedures used most often are coronary artery bypass grafting and coronary angioplasty. These procedures both have been proven to improve symptoms and reduce coronary blockage, diminishing the risk of heart attack. Each has advantages and disadvantages.

Coronary Artery Bypass Grafting

This procedure, also known as bypass surgery, creates a permanent detour around the narrowed or blocked coronary artery or arteries so that blood can reach the heart. This detour is usually created from a leg vein or by linking the internal mammary artery, which carries blood to the chest wall, to the coronary artery. Less commonly, the surgeon may choose to use a forearm artery or the gastroepiploic artery, which supplies blood to the stomach. The choice of procedure and detour material depends on the size of the vessel needed, the number of grafts needed, and a patient's life expectancy (grafts from arteries last longer than grafts from veins), among other considerations.

Coronary artery bypass grafting is major surgery. It involves general anesthesia, an incision in the chest, and, depending on the source of the graft, one or more incisions in the leg, arm, or abdomen. It also involves being attached to a heart-lung bypass machine, which performs the functions of your heart and lungs during the procedure. The procedure usually lasts between three and six hours, depending on the number of bypasses you need. Statistically, the procedure conveys a 2 percent risk of death. The risk jumps to 8 percent if the surgery is performed on an emergency basis, while you're having a heart attack, for example. The risks are highest for people who are older and people who have congestive heart failure. On the positive side, coronary artery bypass grafting can save your life. Indeed, it does so for many people. It also significantly improves symptoms for about 90 percent of patients. Unfortunately, it is not always a permanent solution to the problem. About 40 percent of people who undergo the procedure develop a new blockage within ten years. This underscores the need to make lifestyle modifications in addition to undergoing surgical or medical treatment for ischemic heart disease.

Coronary Angioplasty

In coronary angioplasty, a balloon-tipped catheter is inflated in a narrowed coronary artery to stretch the artery wall and increase its diameter. This procedure is less invasive than bypass surgery, and it generally requires only a local anesthetic. No incision is needed. A guide catheter is inserted into an artery in the groin or arm and threaded to the coronary arteries, guided by X-ray images. A contrast agent or dye is injected into the catheter to make the blockage visible, then a smaller, balloon-tipped catheter is inserted into the guide catheter. When it reaches the blockage, the balloon is inflated, then deflated. The balloon is then removed. In some cases, a stent (a supportive device) may be inserted in the artery to keep the artery open. The entire procedure generally takes between thirty and ninety minutes. It reduces blockage in approximately 95 percent of people and significantly improves symptoms in many.

Though angioplasty is less invasive and less complex than bypass surgery, it is not without possible complications. The insertion of the catheter, for example, can injure an artery, and the balloon inflation can increase the risk of blood clot formation. The risk of death is less than 1 percent. Perhaps more disturbing is the fact that in about one-third of patients, the blockage returns to its original severity in less than a year. As a result, the procedure may have to be repeated or bypass surgery may be needed. In addition, angioplasty may not be appropriate if the blockage is extremely long or if it is in an area that is difficult to reach with a catheter.

MEDICAL

Medical treatments for ischemic heart disease abound. Some are designed to improve heart function, either by promoting blood flow through the coronary arteries or by reducing the heart's demand for oxygen. Others, like aspirin, are designed to reduce the risk of clot formation and heart attack. Often, more than one type of medication is needed. The choice depends in large part on your symptoms. Likewise, your symptoms' reaction to the various medications helps determine whether more high-tech treatment, like angioplasty or bypass surgery, may be needed.

People with mild, infrequent, or predictable angina may be given nitroglycerin pills to take when needed to relieve chest pain or to prevent it after exertion. Nitroglycerin works by dilating, or widening, the blood vessels. This reduces the heart's workload and the heart's demand for oxygen. It also increases the amount of blood that can flow through partially blocked arteries. Longer-term treatments for stable angina may include calcium channel blockers, which reduce heart rate, contraction strength, and blood pressure, thus decreasing the heart's demand for oxygen, and which dilate arteries, thus improving blood flow to the heart; and beta-blockers, which slow the heartbeat and reduce blood pressure and the heart's contraction strength. (I describe the risks and benefits of these medications in the "Hypertension" section.) In addition to one or more of these medications, your treatment may include medication to lower cholesterol levels (see "Cholesterol and Triglyceride Levels") and low-dose aspirin to help prevent clot formation.

Aspirin or another antiplatelet agent is clearly indicated if you have unstable angina. This frequent, intense, or prolonged chest pain is often the result of a triggering of the clotting process. Since unstable angina can easily proceed to heart attack, you will likely be admitted to the hospital where your doctor will try to bring your situation under control and evaluate you to determine if you need to undergo angioplasty or bypass. You may be given one or more of the medications I list above as well as aspirin or another antiplatelet agent. In severe cases, more powerful anticoagulant drugs like heparin or warfarin may be given.

LIFESTYLE

The final component of treating ischemic heart disease, although by no means the least important, involves lifestyle changes that address its underlying cause—atherosclerosis—head on. Our higher-tech treatment options—coronary artery bypass grafting, angioplasty, and medication—address only the results of atherosclerosis; they do not stop its progression. They focus only on one part of the body and do not prevent the redevelopment of atherosclerosis even there. Preliminary research indicates that lifestyle changes can slow or stop the progression of atherosclerosis or, in some cases, even reverse it. These changes include diet, smoking cessation, exercise, and stress reduction.

Diet

A diet high in fat and cholesterol leads to the development of atherosclerotic plaque in the arteries. If you've been diagnosed with ischemic heart disease, you probably already have a buildup. To stop this buildup from progressing—and perhaps reverse it—you should eat a diet that is low in both fat and cholesterol. Research among people with atherosclerosis of the coronary arteries indicates that atherosclerosis can be stopped or reversed with a diet that restricts fat intake to less than 10 percent of total calories and cholesterol intake to less than 5 milligrams per day. Although studies have not yet indicated whether such a diet can reverse atherosclerotic buildup in the carotid arteries, it certainly makes sense to reduce fat and cholesterol intake to those levels, given that you may already be at risk for heart attack. I discuss my dietary recommendations for stroke prevention in detail in the next chapter.

Smoking Cessation

Like diet, smoking contributes to the development and progression of atherosclerosis. If you have been diagnosed with ischemic heart disease, there's a good chance that you already have atherosclerosis. If you smoke, you help the disease progress and increase your risk of both heart attack and ischemic stroke. Regardless of the treatment option or options that you choose, you should seriously consider smoking cessation. I discuss various methods to help you quit on page 169. You should also avoid passive smoke.

Exercise

Physical activity can have profound effects on your cardiovascular (and cerebrovascular) health. First and foremost, it increases your heart's ability to pump blood. It also helps you address heart (and stroke) risk factors, including diabetes mellitus, hypertension, and atherosclerosis. Exercise helps you regulate and control weight, blood sugar, and blood pressure. It may also help you reduce your blood levels of total cholesterol and low-density lipoprotein, which are linked to the development and progression of atherosclerosis. And it can help you reduce stress, which has been linked to an increased risk of heart attack.

If you have ischemic heart disease, you should consult your doctor before launching into an intensive exercise program. Exertion increases your body's demand for oxygen and, depending on the severity of your condition, your heart may not be able to meet that demand. This does not mean that you cannot exercise. It simply means that you will have to start slowly and take it easy. Your cardiologist can help you design a program that can work for—rather than against—your heart.

Stress Reduction

Although some controversy remains, research indicates that stress—and your reaction to it—can increase your risk of heart disease and heart attack. Stress has been proven to increase heart rate and blood pressure. It is known to cause blood vessels to constrict, raise blood sugar levels, and increase the blood's tendency to clot. These responses are particularly troubling if you have ischemic heart disease because they can trigger angina, clot formation, or heart attack. As a result, you need to take steps to reduce stress. Reducing your exposure to stressful situations, learning techniques to cope with those you can't avoid, and practicing relaxation techniques can help you counter these reactions. I detail my suggestions for stress reduction in chapter 5.

Migraine

If you suffer from migraine headaches, particularly those that are preceded by a prodrome, or aura, you are at a very slightly increased risk of ischemic stroke. (Fortunately, the vast majority of people with migraine headaches will not have strokes.) During migraine, the arteries that supply part of the brain constrict in spasm, depriving certain areas of the brain of blood and oxygen—a mechanism similar to that of ischemic stroke. (Ironically, this is not what causes migraine pain. The pain results when arteries outside the skull respond by dilating.) The longer the migraine lasts, the longer the arteries that supply the brain are in spasm, and the greater the risk of ischemic stroke. When it comes to stroke prevention, the goal of treating migraines is to lessen their severity and duration, so that they don't turn into long, potentially dangerous (and extremely painful) episodes. This is done primarily with medications. A doctor familiar with treating migraine can help you determine what medications might work best for you. In addition, you may be able to make certain lifestyle changes to prevent migraine headaches in the first place.

MEDICAL

Medications to treat migraine headaches abound, from aspirin, acetaminophen, and other medications designed primarily to relieve pain, to medications to constrict the extracranial blood vessels, to medications to prevent migraines.

Acute Treatments

Acute treatment for migraine includes analgesics and vasoconstrictors.

Analgesics, which include such standbys as aspirin, acetaminophen (Tylenol), and ibuprofen (Advil) as well as prescription medications, may be effective at relieving mild migraine pain, although they do not address the cause. Many of these medications, like Excedrin, also contain caffeine, which helps reduce pain by constricting the dilated arteries that supply the scalp and cause pain.

Vasoconstrictors work by constricting the extracranial arteries and are among the most commonly prescribed medications for treating moderate and severe migraine. They include sumatriptan (Imitrex), zolmitriptan (Zomig), almotriptan (Axert), naratriptan (Amerge), and rizatriptan; isometheptene, which is found in Midrin; and such ergotamine derivatives as Wigraine, Ergomar, Ergostat, and Cafergot. These drugs are generally most effective when they are taken at the first signs of a migraine. Sumatriptan and related medications have fewer side effects than the other vasoconstrictors and are often effective even when taken well after the migraine attack began. Isometheptene is not recommended for anyone who has glaucoma, severe liver or kidney disease, heart disease, or high blood pressure, because it can worsen these conditions, though it uncommonly causes side effects. Other possible side effects include dizziness and sedation. The ergotamine derivatives, which were commonly prescribed in the past, have taken a secondary role in migraine treatment, because they are less effective than the newer medications and have more side effects. They are not recommended for pregnant or breast-feeding women or people with severe high blood pressure, stomach ulcers, heart problems, vascular disease, or liver or kidney disease. Possible side effects include nausea, vomiting, and itching.

Preventive Medications
If you have debilitating migraines, experience them often, or get no relief from other medications, your doctor may recommend a medication to prevent migraines from occurring. These preventive medications, generally recommended only if you have two or more bad migraines a month that do not respond to treatment, include beta-blockers and calcium channel blockers, antihypertensive medications I discuss in the "Hypertension" section. Beta-blockers prevent migraine by preventing the extracranial arteries from dilating; calcium channel blockers prevent intracranial arteries from contracting. (This prevents the compensatory dilation of extracranial arteries that actually causes the headache.) Other drugs that may help prevent migraine headaches include tricyclic antidepressants and MAO inhibitors,

both of which I discuss in the "Depression" section. These medications stabilize blood levels of serotonin. Shortages of this brain chemical are thought to cause extracranial vascular expansion in a migraine.

LIFESTYLE

In many people, migraine headaches are set off by such triggers as bright or flashing lights, exposure to sunlight, especially at sunrise or sunset, eyestrain, smoking, emotional stress, hormonal changes, hypoglycemia, a change in altitude or weather, or eating certain foods. In many cases, if you know what triggers migraine in you, you may be able to take steps to prevent it.

You may, for example, be able to avoid flashing lights and sunlight. Wear sunglasses and don't look directly at the sun at sunrise and sunset. Avoid smoke. Participate in stress reduction activities. Be aware of hormonal cycles and be aware that oral contraceptives and hormone replacement therapy increase the frequency and severity of migraine attacks. Carry a small snack, and don't go too long without eating if hypoglycemia is a problem. And avoid foods that may trigger headaches. These foods include the following:

Alcohol, especially red wine
Fermented, pickled, or marinated foods
Aged or ripened cheeses (blue, Brie, Camembert, cheddar,
    Emmentaler, Gruyère, Stilton)
Smoked or cured meats (hot dogs, bacon, ham, salami)
Chocolate
Citrus fruits
Nuts, peanut butter
Monosodium glutamate (found in processed and Chinese foods)
Bananas
Pizza
Sourdough bread and other hot, fresh, raised breads
Herring
Chicken livers

You may also want to cut back on or discontinue your caffeine intake. Although caffeine can actually be used to constrict extracranial arteries and relieve migraine pain, the body gets accustomed to it during the day, and temporary withdrawal during the night can trigger headaches in the morning. If you use caffeine, keep your intake at two cups or less per day of a caffeinated beverage.

Mitral or Aortic Heart Valve Disease

Mitral valve stenosis, aortic valve stenosis, severe mitral valve prolapse and other diseases of the mitral and aortic valves can generate clots, which increase the risk of cardioembolic ischemic stroke. Depending on the severity of the problem, mitral or aortic heart valve disease can be treated—and the risk of stroke reduced—by surgery to repair or replace the valves, by medications to reduce the risk of clot formation, or by a combination of both.

SURGICAL/INTERVENTIONAL

A surgical or interventional procedure may be warranted if the valve is seriously damaged. Damaged heart valves can lead to congestive heart failure and rhythm disorders like atrial fibrillation as well as the formation of clots. Depending on the extent of damage, the valve can be repaired or replaced. If it has become narrowed, a catheter procedure called *valvuloplasty* can be used to widen it.

Heart Valve Repair

If your mitral or aortic valve is damaged enough to require surgery or an interventional procedure, your doctor will first determine whether it can be repaired. Repairs generally result in better results and fewer medications. The type of procedure used depends on the type of damage. If the valve leaflets (the parts of the valve that open and close to control blood flow) have become separated from their tethers, for example, the surgeon reconnects them. If the ring of tissue around the base of the valve leaflets is enlarged, the doctor cinches the tissue to tighten it up. The goal is to enable the valve leaflets to close snugly so that blood will not leak. If the valve leaflets have stuck together, causing the valve to narrow and open incompletely, the surgeon may have to cut between them. This procedure is known as *commissurotomy*. These procedures can restore the function of the valve and reduce the risk of clotting and, consequently, ischemic stroke, but they are not without potential complications. They carry such surgical risks as reaction to anesthesia and infection.

Heart Valve Replacement

If the valve is damaged beyond repair, your doctor may recommend replacing it with a mechanical prosthetic valve or with a prosthetic valve made of tissue, from a donor. In either case, the procedure involves removing the damaged valve and replacing it with the new valve. Mechanical heart valves last a long time but increase the risk of clots that could either block the valve or travel to the brain and cause ischemic stroke. As a result, if you have a mechanical heart valve, you will likely need to take an anticoagulant like warfarin for the rest of your life. You may not need anticoagulant therapy if you opt for a tissue heart valve, which does not last as long and may need to be replaced. Regardless of the type of replacement valve you choose, your new valve will be prone to infection. For this reason, you will probably need to take prophylactic antibiotics before you undergo any surgical or dental procedure.

Heart Valvuloplasty

If your mitral or aortic valve is narrowed or obstructed, your doctor may recommend a catheter procedure known as valvuloplasty to open it up. This procedure is similar to angioplasty. A balloon-tipped catheter is threaded through to the heart and inflated to enlarge the valve opening and improve blood flow by separating valve leaflets that have become stuck. The procedure is often preferred over commissurotomy, because it is less invasive. It is not, however, without risk. There is the potential for damage to the valve, and it is not appropriate in all situations—for example, if the calcium buildup on the valve is large, if the valve is allowing blood to leak backward, or if there's a blood clot in one of the heart chambers.

MEDICAL

Mitral and aortic valve diseases can also be treated medically. Depending on the severity of the disease and its effects on your heart's ability to pump, you may need medications to help your heart contract, reduce its workload, or control heart rhythm. These clearly are important, but they play a relatively small role in preventing ischemic stroke. Anticoagulation may also be prescribed. This treatment thins the blood, helps reduce the risk of blood clots, and thus helps to prevent ischemic stroke. Anticoagulants like warfarin (Coumadin) are particularly recommended if the valve problem is complicated by atrial fibrillation, heart failure, or blood clots. The primary side effect of anticoagulants is bleeding or hemorrhage. For people at risk of bleeding, such antiplatelet agents as aspirin or clopidogrel (Plavix) may be beneficial. These drugs also thin the blood, but less effectively. As a result, they do not convey the same risk of bleeding.

Oral Contraceptives/Hormone Replacement

Oral contraceptives and hormone replacement therapy both contain the female hormone estrogen, which appears to have a mixed effect on stroke risk. My interpretation of the research to date is that estrogen increases the risk of the "other" ischemic and cardioembolic ischemic subtypes of stroke but decreases the risk of atherosclerotic ischemic stroke. There appears to be more of an increased risk if you also smoke or have migraine headaches.

If you are a woman at increased risk of atherosclerotic ischemic stroke, you might want to consider using oral contraceptives as your form of birth control or taking hormone replacement during menopause. The estrogen could reduce your risk of this subtype of ischemic stroke. If you are a woman at increased risk of cardioembolic or "other" ischemic stroke, you may want to consider other options.

Patent Foramen Ovale

Patent foramen ovale is a congenital condition in which an opening between the heart's right and left atria (upper chambers) allows a small amount of blood to bypass the lungs. The presence of this opening and the altered blood flow increases the likelihood that clots from the veins will make their way to the brain, causing cardioembolic ischemic stroke. The opening closes soon after birth in most people with the defect. In other people, it remains open to varying degrees or reopens during straining. The severity of the condition dictates treatment. Small openings, or openings that appear only during straining, may simply be monitored. Severe openings may be surgically repaired or treated with such anticoagulants as warfarin (Coumadin, Panwarfin) to prevent the development of clots in the body, for instance, in the legs, which can travel to the heart and through the opening.

Prosthetic Heart Valve

If you have a prosthetic heart valve, particularly a mechanical heart valve, you are at increased risk of generating blood clots. The clots can block the valves or travel through the vascular system to the brain, where they can cause ischemic stroke. To reduce the risk of clot formation—and of stroke—you will likely have to take an anticoagulant like warfarin (Coumadin, Panwarfin) for the rest of your life. Less commonly, you may also be prescribed an antiplatelet agent like aspirin. There is some evidence that the combination further reduces stroke risk. The primary side effect of anticoagulants and, to a lesser extent, antiplatelet agents, is bleeding or hemorrhage.

Recent Heart Attack

Approximately 2 percent of people who suffer heart attacks also suffer ischemic strokes. Most of these strokes occur within the first two weeks after a heart attack. They are typically caused by clots that have formed in the left ventricle. These clots can also be generated by the formation of an aneurysm in the ventricle, a potential complication of heart attack. For these reasons—and the fact that additional clots can develop in the coronary arteries, causing a second heart attack, anticoagulant therapy is commonly given after a heart attack. Therapy often begins with intravenous heparin, then proceeds to oral therapy with warfarin (Coumadin, Panwarfin). This therapy generally lasts for several months. Eventually, it is replaced with long-term antiplatelet therapy.

The primary complication associated with anticoagulants is bleeding. These drugs thin the blood, making it flow more easily. As a result, they increase the risk of hemorrhage. Heparin, the quickest-acting of the anticoagulants, may also lead to the development of thrombocytopenia, in which the number of platelets in the blood is reduced. This condition, too, can prompt bleeding. Antiplatelet agents also thin the blood, although to a lesser extent. As a result, they are less likely to cause hemorrhage than anticoagulants. Aspirin is the best known of these medications. Although it is relatively safe, it can produce such complications as bleeding and gastrointestinal irritation. Others in this class, which may not produce the same side effects, include clopidogrel (Plavix), Aggrenox, a combination of dipyridamole and aspirin, and ticlopidine (Ticlid).

Anticoagulants and antiplatelet agents are crucial in ischemic stroke prevention after heart attack, but they are clearly not the only treatments for heart attack. While the heart attack is in progress, you may be given thrombolytic, or clot-busting, drugs to dissolve the clot in the coronary artery and restore blood flow to the heart. You may also be given such medications as nitroglycerin to improve blood flow through the coronary arteries, and beta-blockers to reduce the workload of the heart and reduce its demand for oxygen. If you have a substantial atherosclerotic blockage in one or more of your coronary arteries, after your condition stabilizes, you may undergo coronary artery bypass grafting or coronary angioplasty to improve blood flow to your heart and prevent future heart attacks. Finally, you and your doctor will address the underlying condition, ischemic heart disease, with lifestyle modifications and, perhaps, additional medications. I discuss these treatments in the "Ischemic Heart Disease" section.

Rheumatic Heart Disease

Rheumatic heart disease is the result of rheumatic fever, an infection that can cause heart inflammation. This infection, caused by certain strains of the streptococcal bacteria, generally begins with an illness common in childhood—strep throat. The infection then moves to the heart, where it often involves the mitral valve and, in many cases, other valves as well. The infection, now relatively uncommon in the United States, is treated with penicillin or another antibiotic. Left untreated, it may cause permanent damage to the heart, particularly damage to the heart valves. This damage may not show up until years after you've recovered from the actual fever. The lasting damage, as well as such complications as atrial fibrillation, increases the risk of clot formation and ischemic stroke, as does the fever itself. The greatest risk occurs within one year after atrial fibrillation begins.

To reduce the risk of stroke, atrial fibrillation and other complications are treated, and severely damaged valves are often repaired or replaced. I discuss these procedures in the sections "Atrial Fibrillation" and "Mitral or Aortic Heart Valve Disease." If rheumatic fever is new and acute, it should be treated with antibiotics, pain relievers, and corticosteroids (to reduce inflammation). Since one bout of rheumatic fever leaves you at greater risk for repeated infection, your doctor will likely recommend long-term antibiotics to prevent reinfection. If the fever first appeared in childhood, antibiotics are generally given until age eighteen. If it first appeared in adulthood, antibiotics are generally given for five years.

Sick Sinus Syndrome

This arrhythmia, which is common among older people, carries the risk of clots and, as a result, of ischemic stroke. We do not yet know with certainty what method of treatment is most appropriate for preventing ischemic stroke in people with sick sinus syndrome who have not experienced a transient ischemic attack or other cerebrovascular event, particularly if the event is felt to be related to sick sinus syndrome. Some experts recommend implantation of a pacemaker; others favor long-term therapy with anticoagulants. However, a pacemaker is generally recommended for people who have had a TIA or minor stroke.

INTERVENTIONAL

If you have sick sinus syndrome, your doctor may recommend a pacemaker. This tiny, battery-operated device is implanted in the chest to do the work of the heart's natural pacemaker and maintain a regular heartbeat. Connected to the heart with flexible leads, it delivers a programmed electrical charge that stimulates the heart to contract. Installation of a pacemaker generally takes about an hour. You are given a local anesthetic; the surgeon makes an incision just below the collarbone, inserts the leads, threads them into your heart, then attaches them to the pacemaker, which is placed in your chest wall. You can generally be discharged from the hospital within one or two days—in some instances, on the same day. Potential side effects include swelling and tenderness, redness, drainage, and fever. Pacemakers generally cause few major complications, but they do eventually wear out. The pacemaker and battery must be monitored regularly to make sure they are still functioning adequately. This can often be done by telephone. When the battery signal becomes weak, you'll need to schedule an appointment to have the pacemaker replaced.

MEDICAL

If you have sick sinus syndrome, your doctor may recommend anticoagulants instead of or in addition to a pacemaker to prevent ischemic stroke. These medications, the most commonly prescribed of which is warfarin

(Coumadin), thin the blood and help reduce the risk of clot formation. Warfarin is generally prescribed as a long-term treatment. The primary side effect of warfarin and other anticoagulants is bleeding or hemorrhage.

Sickle-Cell Disease

Sickle-cell disease can greatly increase the risk of ischemic stroke, particularly in children between the ages of nine and fifteen. This inherited condition, which occurs in about one in six hundred African Americans, causes the red blood cells to become sickle-shaped and clog blood vessels. This generally happens when the blood has too little oxygen. Therefore, the key to ischemic stroke prevention in people with sickle-cell disease is to try to reduce sickling episodes, known as "crises," by maintaining an adequate supply of oxygen. This means avoiding excess physical exertion, dehydration, exposure to excessive heat, infection, or stress, and spending too much time at a high altitude where the oxygen isn't as plentiful, in unpressurized airplanes or the mountains. If the disease does result in cerebrovascular symptoms, your doctor might recommend transfusions of healthy red blood cells to prevent stroke.

Smoking

If you're a smoker, you know what I'm going to tell you: Stop. You also know that that's easier said than done. If you can quit cold turkey, by all means do so. Quitting significantly reduces your risk of ischemic and hemorrhagic stroke. Numerous other health benefits also await you, but I'm sure you know this. You also know that nicotine is extremely addictive, and you may need help to break the addiction. Fortunately, help is available—in many forms. You are likely to find one or more methods or aids that work for you—particularly if you seek professional help. A smoking or nicotine dependence center in a hospital or medical center near you can assess your dependence, direct you to the method or methods that are most likely to succeed for you as an individual, and provide you with needed support. Of course, you can also try one or more methods or aids on your own. Methods and aids include medications, counseling, and numerous lifestyle efforts. Your doctor or a smoking cessation specialist can help you find a method that is likely to work for you.

MEDICAL

Medical treatments for smoking cessation are designed primarily to help you cope with nicotine withdrawal. They do one of two things: replace the nicotine you would normally get in cigarettes, allowing you gradually to wean yourself from the drug, or act in another way to reduce nicotine cravings. These medications have been shown significantly to increase rates of quitting when they are included as part of an intervention program, but they are not panaceas. They are less effective when they are used alone, and they are to be used only for the short term.

Nicotine Replacement

The primary medical treatment for smoking cessation is nicotine replacement. This short-term therapy prevents such nicotine withdrawal symptoms as cravings, irritability, anxiety, and restlessness, by replacing the nicotine you would normally get from cigarettes. It helps you gradually reduce your intake of and craving for nicotine. Nicotine replacement comes in several forms and doses. The transdermal patch delivers a steady dose of nicotine through the skin. The dose is gradually reduced. Four brands of nicotine patches are currently available. Habitrol and Prostep require a doctor's prescription; Nicoderm and Nicotrol are available over the counter. Nicotine gum, sold over the counter as Nicorette, delivers nicotine through the lining of the mouth. Its absorption may be affected if you put anything else in your mouth while you are using it. Nicotine nasal spray, available only by prescription, delivers the nicotine directly to the bloodstream, through the lining of the nose. For this reason, it may relieve withdrawal symptoms more quickly than the patch or gum. The final aid, the nicotine inhaler, delivers nicotine through the mouth when you inhale, much as a cigarette does. In fact, it resembles a cigarette in size and shape.

Nicotine replacement can be very helpful, but only if the person actually stops smoking and follows recommendations for tapering off and, eventually, ceasing treatment. You need to bear in mind that while you are taking a nicotine replacement medication, you are still delivering nicotine to your body. Although you are getting it in a lower dose and a healthier fashion than you would through cigarette smoking, it is still an unhealthy, addictive drug.

Buproprion

Another type of medication prescribed for smoking cessation is buproprion (Zyban), an antidepressant that has been found to reduce nicotine cravings. It is believed to work by stimulating the release of dopamine, a brain chemical that causes a positive response similar to that produced by nicotine. Buproprion is nonaddictive and does not contain nicotine, but it has potential side effects. These include agitation, dry mouth, insomnia, headache, nausea, vomiting, constipation, and tremor.

LIFESTYLE

Lifestyle modifications constitute the bulk of methods and aids for smoking cessation. After all, smoking is a lifestyle choice. So is smoking cessation. It is a conscious change in behavior. From making a list of motivating reasons to quit, to preparing ways to address nicotine addiction, to entering into counseling, you are taking action to change your behavior and your life. As you can see from those examples, some lifestyle methods can be tackled alone, others require outside help.

Motivation

This is perhaps the most important factor in smoking cessation. Although motivation to stop smoking may not lead to success on its own, without it, you're doomed to failure. This is true whether you enter a formal treatment program or design your own method or program. Most treatment programs and self-help programs recommend that you begin by deciding that you want to quit and determining why. They often suggest that you make a list of reasons to quit: for your health, for your family, to save money. They may suggest that you review the various health problems caused by smoking, that you prepare yourself to quit by learning all that you can about the various withdrawal symptoms you may face as well as ways to cope. There's no arguing with this approach. It's a logical, necessary first step to changing your behavior.

Motivation is also important as you proceed with whatever method you choose to stop smoking, and it can play a role in keeping you tobacco free. After you stop smoking, give yourself at least a month or so to see how much better you feel. This can be a big motivator in staying away from cigarettes.

STROKE - FREE for LIFE

Coping Techniques

Whether you tackle smoking cessation on your own or as part of a formal program, you will need to amass a set of coping techniques to help you deal with nicotine withdrawal. The techniques you choose, obviously, will depend on the symptoms you experience as well as on your individual preferences. To reduce nicotine cravings, for example, you may try to distract yourself or do deep breathing exercises. To counter insomnia, you may want to avoid caffeine, take a warm bath, or exercise several hours before bedtime. The list of possible techniques is virtually endless. Organizations like the American Cancer Society and American Lung Association provide information on coping techniques, as do many formal smoking cessation programs. You can also ask your doctor for advice or ask friends and family members what worked for them. Not every technique will work for you, and you may not need help in certain areas. You may find that these techniques, combined with motivation, can be helpful, if not necessary, in accomplishing your goal.

Support Groups

Regardless of whether you are quitting on your own or participating in a formal smoking cessation program, support groups are often helpful. It can help you to know that others are going or have gone through the same experiences you are undergoing. They can give you advice, encouragement, and support and help you stay focused on your goal.

Counseling

Counseling, in an individual or group setting, may be able to provide you with the motivation, support, and coping techniques you need to stop smoking. Many smoking cessation programs offer a choice of individual or group counseling. In either case, counseling can help you understand why you smoke, teach you to change your behavior, help you cope with the changes you are making, and provide support. Many of these programs include discussions of the medical aspects of smoking, coping skills, stress management, and relapse prevention.

Hypnosis

Hypnosis is a state of mind in which relaxation is enhanced and focus and suggestibility are heightened. When you are hypnotized, you can be directed to perceive things differently and think about possibilities you haven't thought about before. This can be helpful if you're trying to quit smoking. A psychologist can direct you in using the power of your mind to cope with nicotine withdrawal symptoms. This does not mean your mind will be controlled. Hypnosis can't make you do anything that you don't really want to do. Not all people can be hypnotized. Some, particularly those who don't want to feel that they may be out of control, are unable to go into a hypnotic state or trance.

Residential Treatment Programs

If your addiction is severe, you may benefit from an intensive residential treatment program like the one we offer at the Mayo Nicotine Dependence Center. These inpatient programs are offered in a tobacco-free setting that is supervised to prevent participants from lighting up. They generally include individual and group counseling, medical treatment for nicotine withdrawal, educational sessions about the effects of smoking, stress management, and other pertinent topics, and physician supervision.

Stimulant Drugs

Drugs that produce rapid, temporary spikes in blood pressure—including caffeine—may increase the risk of intracerebral hemorrhage or rupture of intracranial aneurysms or vascular malformations in the brain, which, in turn, increases the risk of hemorrhagic stroke. If you know or suspect you have an intracranial aneurysm or vascular malformation, you should talk with your doctor or pharmacist about the medications you are taking—prescription or nonprescription. If any are known to cause rapid increases in blood pressure, a substitution may be in order. If you suffer from allergies, for example, you may be able to take an antihistamine like diphenhydramine (Benadryl) rather than a decongestant like pseudoephedrine.

Consider cutting back on caffeine as well. Although we're more likely to think of caffeine as a food additive, it is also a drug. Regardless of whether we ingest caffeine for pleasure or as an ingredient of over-the-counter medication, it can cause temporary spikes in blood pressure and, thus, has the potential to increase the risk of aneurysm or vascular malformation rupture. Cutting back your daily caffeine intake to the amount in two caffeinated beverages—or avoiding it altogether—could reduce your risk of hemorrhagic stroke.

Stress

Stress can increase blood pressure—either temporarily, which can increase the risk of aneurysm or vascular malformation rupture, as well as the risk of intracerebral hemorrhage, or chronically, which can also increase your risk of intracerebral hemorrhage. Overall, stress increases the risk of hemorrhagic stroke and atherosclerotic and lacunar ischemic stroke. It can affect other aspects of your health as well. Unfortunately, it's virtually impossible to avoid stress completely in today's world. Lifestyle changes and, in extreme cases, medications can make it possible to reduce stress and relieve its effects.

MEDICAL

Although I believe that medical treatment of stress should be a last resort—lifestyle techniques can be equally or more effective and carry fewer side effects—there is a place for medication (particularly short-term) in the treatment of severe stress and anxiety. The drugs include antidepressants, antianxiety drugs, sedatives, and sleep aids.

Antidepressants

Many antidepressants, including tricyclic antidepressants, monoamine oxidase inhibitors, and selective serotonin reuptake inhibitors, can be used to treat stress. These medications work by changing the balance of certain brain chemicals, which affect mood. They are discussed in more detail in the section on "Depression" earlier in this chapter.

Benzodiazepines

These drugs, which include Librium, Xanax, Valium, Dalmane, and Halcion, like the antidepressants, work by enhancing the activities of certain brain chemicals and inhibiting others. They are usually recommended only for short-term (two weeks or less) or sporadic treatment, largely because they can be addictive. They can also cause drowsiness and affect coordination.

Beta-Blockers

These antihypertensive medications also have a stress-reducing effect. They block the brain's beta waves, which are associated with the stress hormone epinephrine or adrenaline. I discuss these drugs in detail in the "Hypertension" section.

Sleep Aids

Getting a good night's sleep is a good way to relieve stress. Likewise, insomnia can be stressful. Prescription and over-the-counter sleep aids can help combat sleeplessness, including some of the tranquilizing drugs mentioned above. For occasional insomnia due to stress, I believe over-the-counter remedies like melatonin or Benadryl are preferable. Melatonin is a naturally occurring brain chemical; Benadryl is an antihistamine that has sedating effects. These options are less apt to cause dependence than prescription sleep aids. Incidentally, if insomnia is a problem for you, you should drink no more than two cups of coffee or other caffeinated beverage a day and avoid drinking caffeinated beverages with or after dinner. You should also do any exercise before dinner rather than before bedtime.

LIFESTYLE

Lifestyle changes are the hallmark of stress reduction. From simplifying and organizing your life to exercising to performing relaxation techniques, lifestyle changes can help you reduce the amount of stress you face and cope with what remains. This can make you happier and healthier, as well as reduce your risk of hemorrhagic stroke. I discuss strategies to reduce stress in detail in the next chapter.

Transient Ischemic Attack/Minor Ischemic Stroke

If you've experienced a transient ischemic attack, reversible ischemic neurologic deficit (RIND), or minor ischemic stroke, you clearly need to take action to reduce your risk of experiencing a major ischemic stroke. This is particularly true if the event occurred recently or if you also have a condition that increases the likelihood of clot formation. Fortunately, you have a number of treatment options from which to choose, ranging from surgery and medications to lifestyle changes. In many cases, the right prescription for you may include various options in combination.

SURGICAL/INTERVENTIONAL

Carotid endarterectomy is the surgical procedure that probably comes to your mind as a treatment for transient ischemic attack. It is the most commonly performed surgical procedure for ischemic stroke prevention, although it is not the only option. Others include carotid angioplasty and rarely artery-

artery bypass. These procedures are designed to reduce narrowing, open up a blockage, or reroute blood around a narrowing or blockage in the arteries that supply blood to the brain.

Carotid Endarterectomy

This procedure, developed in the 1950s, is among the most commonly performed operations in the United States. In the early 1980s, it was second only to cataract surgery among Medicare patients. Despite its popularity, carotid endarterectomy is not always appropriate. The procedure—in which the surgeon makes an incision in the neck, clamps off the carotid artery, opens the artery, scrapes off the atherosclerotic plaque on the artery's inner lining, then closes the artery and removes the clamps (see figure, page 108)—can significantly reduce ischemic stroke risk in certain people, particularly those who have experienced symptoms within the past four months. In fact, studies indicate that the procedure can reduce the risk of ischemic stroke from 26 to 7 percent over two years in people with severe narrowing of the carotid artery causing TIA or minor ischemic stroke. In other people, the procedure can have little or no effect on ischemic stroke risk. What's more, it has the potential to actually trigger ischemic stroke and heart attack, and, less commonly, hemorrhagic stroke. Other surgical complications, including reaction to the anesthetic, infection, and scarring, are also possible. You must seriously consider these risks—as well as the potential benefits of the procedure—before you decide on this option.

Fortunately, data accumulated from randomized trials of carotid endarterectomy offer clear insight into who might benefit from the procedure—and who might not. Although the procedure can theoretically be performed on anyone who has stenosis, or narrowing, of the carotid artery, it is generally most beneficial to patients who have experienced symptoms— TIA, or minor ischemic stroke (including RIND) qualify if caused by a lesion in the carotid artery—and who have a significant narrowing of the corresponding carotid. Research indicates that you are most likely to benefit from the procedure if you have experienced symptoms and if the diameter of your carotid artery is reduced by 70 percent or more. You also may benefit if you have experienced symptoms and the diameter of your carotid artery is reduced by 50 to 69 percent. You are unlikely to benefit if the narrowing of your carotid artery reduces its diameter by less than 50 percent.

If you have severe or progressive kidney, liver, or heart disease, a cancer with a low survival rate, another condition that may generate cerebral embolism or clots, or you have uncontrolled diabetes mellitus or uncontrolled hypertension, your doctor will have to weigh the risks and benefits of the procedure in view of your individual situation. Your overall health should also be a consideration, as should the choice of a surgeon. Each of these factors can increase the risk of complications from carotid endarterectomy. If your risk of stroke is even higher—say, you have significant narrowing of your artery and your doctor has identified an ulcer or clot—the benefits of the procedure may be more likely to outweigh the risks.

Because of the risk involved in carotid endarterectomy, it should be performed only by an experienced surgeon with a low rate of complications and death. If you opt for this procedure, I recommend that you find a surgeon with a combined complication and death rate for the procedure of less than 6 percent on patients with symptoms and less than 3 percent on patients without symptoms. These rates are often difficult to accurately determine, in large part because some surgeons may not have performed the procedure often enough to ensure statistical validity. Although some states are collecting these data, not all are. Ask your surgeon for any published data he or she might have.

Carotid Artery Angioplasty

Another surgical option for treating TIA, RIND, or minor ischemic stroke and reducing the risk of major ischemic stroke is carotid angioplasty. Although this procedure, in which a balloon-tipped catheter is threaded through the blood vessels into the blocked carotid artery, then inflated to open the artery and facilitate blood flow, is being used in some medical centers, it is still considered experimental. Its effectiveness has not yet been adequately compared to that of carotid endarterectomy, and nobody knows in what instances it will prove to be preferable. That said, the procedure does have some apparent advantages—local, rather than general anesthesia, the lack of an incision, and, generally, an expectation of a shorter recovery period and hospital stay. There are some instances when it might be considered, for example, if you have a condition that increases the risk of open surgery, but you are otherwise a candidate for carotid endarterectomy, or if the technical aspects of approaching the artery in an open procedure are extremely difficult. Carotid angioplasty is not without potential complications. It can result in dissection or rupture of the carotid artery or the formation of an aneurysm, embolism, or blood vessel blockage. At this point, carotid angioplasty is not widely recommended or widely available. Angioplasty may also be performed on blockages in other intracranial arteries, although again, the procedure is not widespread.

Extracranial-Intracranial Bypass

Another surgical option available for people who have had a TIA, RIND, or minor ischemic stroke is extracranial-to-intracranial bypass. This procedure, which involves the diversion of blood from one of the external arteries supplying structures outside the skull to an internal artery, was once widely performed to prevent ischemic stroke. The results of a major study published in 1985 found that it is generally ineffective as a stroke preventive. There are some rare instances when this procedure may be useful. If a large aneurysm or tumor is blocking or invading an artery, for example, the sacrifice of the artery may help prevent ischemic stroke. The procedure may also be recommended if a blockage or high-grade narrowing of an artery is causing repeated, incapacitating TIAs or progressive visual loss.

MEDICAL

Medication, in the form of anticoagulants or antiplatelet agents, is a standard stroke preventive for people who have experienced TIAs, RINDs, or minor ischemic strokes. It may be given as immediate treatment for the event itself; it may be the primary form of long-term prevention if surgery is not an option; and it may be given as a long-term preventive after surgery.

Depending on your personal situation, medical treatment may also include drugs to treat diabetes and/or hypertension. These conditions commonly occur in conjunction with atherosclerosis and are known to exacerbate it. There is some evidence that both hypertension and atherosclerosis are the result of problems in the endothelial tissue, the layer of cells that line internal organs.

Anticoagulants

In many cases, treatment for a TIA or minor ischemic stroke begins with the anticoagulant drug warfarin for three to six months, followed by long-term treatment with an antiplatelet agent like aspirin or clopidogrel. If your risk of major ischemic stroke is extremely high—say, you've had more than four TIAs in the past two weeks, or you have atrial fibrillation or a mechanical heart valve—your treatment may begin with intravenous heparin, then progress to warfarin and, eventually, to an antiplatelet agent.

The primary complication associated with anticoagulants is bleeding. These drugs thin the blood, making it flow more easily. As a result, they increase the risk of intracerebral hemorrhage, especially in people with chronic high blood pressure. This is most common with heparin, the quickest-acting of the anticoagulants. Heparin may also lead to the development of thrombocytopenia, in which the number of platelets in the blood is reduced. This condition, too, can prompt bleeding. Because of these complications, heparin should be used to treat TIAs only if the risk of major ischemic stroke is very high. The risk of bleeding is lower with warfarin, particularly with lower dosages. As with heparin, high blood pressure may increase the risk. Age may have the same effect.

Antiplatelet Agents

Antiplatelet agents also thin the blood, although to a lesser extent. These medications, which include aspirin, dipyridamole (Persantine), clopidogrel (Plavix), Aggrenox, a combination of dipyridamole and aspirin, and ticlopidine (Ticlid), may be prescribed as initial treatment for TIA or ischemic stroke, especially if there is no evidence of significant narrowing of the carotid artery. They can also be prescribed as a long-term preventive following other treatments.

Research indicates that people who take aspirin after a previous stroke or TIA reduce their risk of ischemic stroke by approximately 20 percent. The dosage typically ranges from 80 milligrams a day to 650 milligrams twice a day. This simple, inexpensive medication clearly plays a major role in stroke prevention. Though aspirin is relatively safe, it can produce complications like bleeding and gastrointestinal irritation. The risk of these complications is lower with lower doses. Still, there are people who cannot take aspirin because of these side effects or because of an allergy. These people may benefit from one of the newer antiplatelet agents. These medications are more expensive than aspirin, but they may be slightly more effective. One study, for instance, found that ticlopidine is 10 percent more effective than aspirin in reducing ischemic stroke risk but causes more side effects. Another found that clopidogrel is 8.8 percent more effective; however, a recent review indicates that clopidogrel's advantage is primarily among people with peripheral arterial disease, atherosclerosis of peripheral arteries, like those that deliver blood to the arms and legs.

Effectiveness may also be increased by combining aspirin with another antiplatelet agent. In a large study published in 1996, the combination of aspirin and dipyridimole almost doubled the reduction in stroke risk of aspirin alone—37 percent versus 21 percent. Approximately three years later, the U.S. Food and Drug Administration approved a new drug, Aggrenox, that combines the two antiplatelet agents.

LIFESTYLE

Lifestyle changes that address the development and progression of atherosclerosis—the underlying cause of most instances of artery narrowing—are among the best ways to treat TIA and minor ischemic stroke. Unlike the other treatments I discuss, they target atherosclerosis all over the body, and they do it in a natural way. Every medication and surgical procedure has some side effect or risk, but lifestyle changes like a healthy diet, smoking cessation, and stress reduction do not. In fact, they offer health benefits other than simply treating atherosclerosis. I strongly recommend that you opt for these changes when you design your prescription, regardless of the medical or surgical treatments you choose.

Diet

A diet high in fat and cholesterol leads to the development of atherosclerotic plaque in the arteries. If you've had a TIA or minor ischemic stroke, chances are good that it was caused by atherosclerosis, and you already have a buildup. To stop this buildup from progressing—and potentially even reverse it—you should eat a diet that is very low in both saturated fat and cholesterol. Research among people with atherosclerosis of the coronary arteries indicates that atherosclerosis can be stopped or reversed with a diet that restricts fat intake to less than 10 percent of total calories and cholesterol intake to less than 5 milligrams per day. Although studies have not yet indicated whether such a diet can reverse atherosclerotic buildup in the carotid arteries, I believe it makes sense to reduce fat and cholesterol intake to somewhat comparable levels. The typical American gets approximately 40 percent of his or her calories from fat and takes in 400 milligrams of cholesterol a day. If you are really serious about treating—or reversing—atherosclerosis, you have to do much more than follow the "healthy diet" guidelines recommended by the federal government and many health organizations. These guidelines, which restrict fat intake to no more than 30 percent of total calories and cholesterol intake to no more than 300 milligrams of cholesterol a day, are not very effective. I believe we need to go further. I discuss my dietary recommendations in detail in the next chapter.

Smoking Cessation

Like diet, smoking contributes to the development and progression of atherosclerosis. If you have had a TIA or minor ischemic stroke, there's a good chance that you already have atherosclerosis. If you smoke, you help the disease progress and increase your risk of having a major ischemic stroke. Regardless of the treatment option or options that you choose, you should seriously consider smoking cessation. I discuss various methods to help you quit on page 169.

Stress Reduction

The link between stress and atherosclerosis is an indirect one, but I believe stress reduction plays a role in bringing atherosclerosis under control—or preventing its development. Stress is known to increase blood pressure, and high blood pressure has been linked to atherosclerosis. In fact, the two often go hand in hand. For suggestions on how to decrease your stress level, see page 174 and chapter 5.

Vascular Malformations

Intracranial vascular malformations, like intracranial aneurysms, have the potential to rupture, causing hemorrhagic stroke. And although the surgical procedures used to treat these abnormalities differ from those used to treat aneurysms, the medical and lifestyle procedures to reduce the risk of rupture and, subsequently, the risk of hemorrhagic stroke, are much the same.

SURGICAL/INTERVENTIONAL

As with intracranial aneurysms, the risk of rupture and the patient's condition play major roles in the choice of surgery or conservative treatment for vascular malformation. Total removal is generally the preferred surgical treatment whenever possible, but other procedures, including embolization and radiotherapy, may be used—alone or in combination—to isolate the malformation from its blood supply without physically removing it.

Removal

Total surgical removal is the most thorough treatment for vascular malformation. It removes the malformation, which removes the threat of rupture and significantly reduces the risk of hemorrhagic stroke. However, total removal is not always possible. The size, type, or location of the malformation may make it difficult or even impossible to remove. The patient's physical condition and age may increase the risks of the procedure. Or an experienced neurosurgeon may not be available. This is a technical procedure that should be performed only by a skilled specialist.

Generally speaking, the procedure is most beneficial for young, healthy patients whose malformations are of a size and location that makes removal relatively safe. This includes both people who have experienced symptoms and those who have not. The risk of hemorrhage is about 2 percent a year even in people who do not experience symptoms. The overall risk to the patient is higher if neurologic symptoms are progressing, if seizures become unmanageable, or if the malformation begins to bleed. The best candidates for surgical removal are those who have a small arteriovenous malformation (AVM) in the frontal or temporal area of the brain.

Surgical removal may not be possible for large AVMs, especially those that involve more than one area of the brain, and for AVMs located deep in the brain in a high-risk area. This is, after all, brain surgery. It carries the risk of death and complications as well as such standard surgical risks as infection and reaction to anesthesia. In fact, surgery for AVMs located deep in the brain or in another high-risk area carries a complication rate of 10 to 25 percent, including a death rate of 1 to 5 percent.

Endovascular Embolization

Embolization is a procedure to block or reduce blood flow. Endovascular embolization is a procedure to block or reduce blood flow through vessels; in this case, through the vessels that feed the malformation. Any of a number of substances may be used to cut off the blood flow—from glue to muscle. Embolization may precede or follow surgical removal of the malformation, particularly if several large blood vessels supply the malformation. Although it can be used alone, it rarely is used as a sole treatment for AVMs, because the long-term effectiveness of the various embolization materials is unknown. It is often used in conjunction with surgery or radiotherapy.

Radiotherapy

Radiotherapy, or radiation therapy, can be used alone or with embolization to treat vascular malformations that are inoperable. Focused forms, such as gamma knife radiotherapy and proton beam radiation, are among the most high-tech. Gamma knife radiotherapy is a form of radiation so precise that it acts like a surgical tool. Guided by a computer, this procedure involves the delivery of a three-dimensional beam of radiation to a precise target, for example the nidus, or center, of a vascular malformation that cannot be removed. This causes the lining of the vascular walls to enlarge, which eventually closes the malformation, cutting it off from the circulation. Gamma knife radiotherapy and other focused types of radiation therapy can obliterate the malformation, but they take some time. In 40 percent of cases, the malformation is gone one year after treatment; in approximately 80 percent, it is gone after two years; and in more than 90 percent, it is gone after three years. However, while it remains, it presents a risk of hemorrhage.

Gamma knife radiotherapy is particularly effective for smaller AVMs, those in which the nidus is 2 centimeters in diameter or less. Radiotherapy alone is not an optimum treatment for AVMs that are more than 3 centimeters in diameter.

MEDICAL

Although no medications are available to treat intracranial vascular malformations or to prevent them from rupturing, medications that sharply increase blood pressure may increase the risk of rupture. If you have a vascular malformation, you should talk with your doctor or pharmacist about any medications you are taking—prescription or nonprescription. If any are known to cause rapid increases in blood pressure, a substitution may be in order.

In addition, you should avoid anticoagulants and antiplatelet agents. Although these drugs do not necessarily cause vascular malformations to rupture, they can make a rupture worse.

LIFESTYLE

If you are not a candidate for surgery, you can make lifestyle changes that reduce your risk of rapidly increasing your blood pressure and, thus, reduce your risk of malformation rupture. This, in turn, reduces your risk of both subarachnoid hemorrhage and intracerebral hemorrhage.

Stress Reduction

Stress is known to spike blood pressure, and there is some evidence that temporary, rapid increases in blood pressure may cause a vascular malformation to rupture. For these reasons, if you have a vascular malformation, it's wise to pay attention to your stress level and take steps to reduce it as much as possible. Stress reduction has other benefits as well. I discuss stress reduction in detail in chapter 5.

Straining Avoidance

As I've said, rapid spikes in blood pressure may increase the risk of aneurysm rupture. Although day-to-day exercise and activities do not appear to be a problem, activities that cause you to strain can produce these spikes. If you have an unruptured aneurysm, you should think twice before performing such activities. Don't try to move furniture by yourself, for example. Use a stool softener if constipation causes you to strain. And make your exercise aerobic rather than isometric.

Caffeine Avoidance

Caffeine is present in our coffee, our soft drinks, our chocolate, and our pain relievers. It's one of our most widely used drugs. When we ingest caffeine, it causes a temporary spike in blood pressure, and thus has the potential to increase the risk of aneurysm rupture. Cutting back your caffeine intake to two cups a day or less of a caffeinated beverage—or avoiding it altogether—could reduce your risk of hemorrhagic stroke.

Alcohol Avoidance

Alcohol consumption, particularly heavy alcohol consumption and binge drinking, has been linked to both types of hemorrhagic stroke. If you drink heavily or binge drink, you should consider reducing your alcohol intake or avoiding alcohol altogether. I discuss ways to reduce alcohol consumption in the "Alcohol" section on page 97.

Ventricular Aneurysm

Ventricular aneurysm is an expansion, or ballooning, of the wall of one of the heart's ventricles. These aneurysms generally appear after a heart attack and can spark the development of clots that can make their way to the brain, causing ischemic stroke. This condition is not an easy one to treat. Often, the preferred course of action is to simply leave it alone and monitor the area for the development of clots. If a clot occurs, it can be surgically removed or treated with anticoagulants. (See the "Clot in Heart" section on page 127 for more information.) If the aneurysm poses additional risks, it can be treated surgically. The procedure involves trying to cut away the excess ventricular wall and re-forming the heart. This procedure is not without risks.

You now have the information you need to develop a personalized prescription for stroke prevention. But stroke prevention doesn't end with treating existing risk factors. It's an ongoing lifestyle commitment to keeping your risk level low and preventing new risk factors from developing—which amounts to a brain-healthy lifestyle. In the next chapter, I outline a program based on diet, exercise, and stress management that can further reduce your risk of stroke, regardless of your current risk level, and keep it low for life.

5

The Stroke-Free for Life Prevention Plan

If you're at low risk for stroke, congratulations. In this chapter, I offer you a plan to stay low-risk for life. It's not based on medications—though if you're not at low risk, you may need to supplement this plan with medication. Rather, it incorporates a menu of brain-healthy lifestyle habits that can keep your risk of stroke low for as long as you stay on it.

It's a plan "for life" in two respects:

- It's life-centered. All the aspects of this plan will enhance not only your longevity but also your overall health and vitality—which will also increase your enjoyment of daily life.
- It's a sustainable, long-term plan that you can stay with for years, rather than weeks or months.

I'm not saying that lifestyle adaptations are easy. I'm always impressed, for instance, by how deep-seated our dietary habits are, physically and emotionally. The reason this plan is sustainable over a long period of time is that it's a self-reinforcing program—the immediate and ongoing rewards will be your primary impetus for staying on the plan. The better you feel from a healthy lifestyle, the more motivated you'll be to stay healthy.

Your stroke prevention prescription should be tailored to fit your unique risk profile. Regardless of whether your profile puts you at high, medium, or low risk, lifestyle choices should be a major part of that prescription. Lifestyle choices—what to eat, how much to exercise, how to reduce stress—are powerful life-changing tools. If you use them to your advantage, you can significantly reduce your risk of stroke or keep it low. Best of all, these tools, which form the building blocks of my Stroke-Free for Life Plan, are completely within your control.

If you're at high or medium risk of stroke, lifestyle changes may already be a part of your prescription, particularly if you have atherosclerosis, hypertension, or diabetes mellitus. These conditions can be controlled—in some cases, completely—with diet, exercise, and stress reduction. Even if you do not have one of these chronic conditions, you can benefit from adopting brain-healthy habits. Anything you can do to prevent additional risk factors from developing can have a positive effect on your overall stroke risk, which is why I recommend lifestyle changes even for people who are at low risk of stroke. Over time, the development of various conditions and, of course, aging can alter the picture. Though there's not much you can do to stop the clock, you can take steps to slow the physical aging process, prevent the development of certain conditions, and keep your risk of stroke low.

The Stroke-Free for Life Plan is primarily a lifestyle plan. It consists of healthy diet—including foods that may offer protection against stroke—regular physical exercise, and stress reduction. Anyone can benefit from the healthy habits I outline in this chapter, from the eighty-year-old man with hypertension and ischemic heart disease to the healthy thirty-year-old woman with no stroke risk factors. The basic principles are similar for everybody. Tastes, preferences, and physical abilities figure into the prescription just as age and weight figure into the dosage of a prescribed medication. The guidelines are easy to follow, inexpensive, and accessible.

In addition to reducing your risk of stroke, the lifestyle changes in the Stroke-Free for Life Plan can help you lower your risk of hypertension, ischemic heart disease, diabetes, and cancer. They will give you added energy, improve your physical strength and flexibility, boost your immunity, and give you peace of mind. In other words, this plan is a win-win proposition.

Although lifestyle choices are the primary tools of the Stroke-Free for Life Plan, some people may gain additional benefits from medications. Although medications are primarily used to treat the chronic conditions that increase stroke risk, in some cases they may offer independent protection or, even more exciting, possibly prevent certain risk factors from developing.

HEALTHY LIFESTYLE: THE KEY TO TRULY PREVENTING STROKE

It's no secret that unhealthy lifestyle choices we make can lead to the development of stroke risk factors. A lifetime of smoking, eating high-fat foods, and being sedentary can set you up for atherosclerosis, ischemic heart disease, hypertension, and diabetes mellitus. Changing these unhealthy habits is a major part of controlling these conditions and keeping them from progressing. If you make those lifestyle changes earlier—before these conditions develop—the beneficial effect can be even greater. Lifestyle changes become the ultimate stroke prevention tool by preventing the development of the diseases that cause stroke. If you avoid tobacco, follow a healthy diet, avoid alcohol or drink alcohol only in moderation, exercise, and take action to reduce the stress in your life, you can reduce your risk of ever having a stroke as well as your risk of atherosclerosis, diabetes mellitus, hypertension, ischemic heart disease, and cancer.

Unfortunately, many people in the medical community view lifestyle changes more as a stroke treatment, or a means to prevent a second stroke, than as a primary stroke preventive. This is an ineffective and outdated perspective. If we have the vision to prescribe and promote healthy lifestyles, we can prevent stroke, as well as most of the other leading causes of death and disability. If you're at low risk for stroke, I urge you to seize this opportunity to give yourself the longest possible life with the fullest function. What do you have to lose?

Diet
Diet can help prevent stroke in two ways: It can prevent the development or progression of such stroke risk factors as atherosclerosis, hypertension, ischemic heart disease, diabetes mellitus, and a high cholesterol level, and it can provide beneficial nutrients and food components that can independently reduce stroke risk as well as the risk of other diseases. My diet plan takes both of these factors into account, offering general guidelines for such

major food components as fat and cholesterol as well as a list of foods and supplements that may offer additional protection.

MY DIETARY PRINCIPLES

Before I outline my diet plan, I'd like to explain the principles behind it. Food is the fuel that keeps our bodies running. It can also be a major source of health or a major source of illness. If we eat the right foods, we can enhance our health. If we eat the wrong foods, we can develop fatal illnesses. In choosing what to eat, I believe we should look at what foods are healthful and what foods are harmful for our overall health. As a neurologist, I also look at what foods are good for the brain and cerebrovascular system. Some of this information is easy to find. For example, research has shown that a diet high in fat and cholesterol can lead to the development of atherosclerosis, which is a risk factor for ischemic stroke as well as ischemic heart disease.

This does not mean that we should chase after every new theory, study, or diet that is introduced. If we did, our diet would change dramatically from day to day, and we might be eating unhealthily as often as we are eating healthily. Conflicting reports abound about the health benefits of many foods—and of overall diets.

Speaking of diets, anyone who tries to lose weight by dieting alone clearly risks following questionable eating advice. For instance, some fad weight-loss diets have promoted the idea of eating simply cabbage or simply grapefruit. Neither diet could be considered healthy, although both foods are healthy in and of themselves. We simply weren't meant to eat only one type of food. No one food contains all the nutrients our bodies need.

The latest popular diets—those that greatly restrict carbohydrates—also have me concerned. Many of these diets are based on the theory that a diet high in carbohydrates causes the body to increase insulin levels, causing the pancreas to work harder and, eventually, leading to insulin resistance. Insulin resistance, in turn, can cause the body to store fat and, possibly, to develop diabetes mellitus.

The theory holds that a low-carbohydrate diet, particularly a diet low in simple carbohydrates that rapidly turn to glucose and raise levels of blood sugar, will help the body lose weight. Low-carbohydrate diets do cause weight loss. When you stop eating carbohydrates—the body's primary source of fuel—your body rather quickly begins depleting its stores of glycogen (starch) to provide the blood with glucose (a form of sugar). Glycogen is stored in water, so when it is burned, water weight is also lost. This often results in the quick drop of four or six pounds. Eventually, the body must burn protein and fat to obtain glucose. Neither of these options is ideal. For starters, the body needs some protein for a variety of functions, including as a building block for muscle and skin. For another, the breakdown of protein, which contains nitrogen, results in the production of ammonia, a toxic product the body converts to the slightly less toxic waste product urea, which must be cleared from the body by the kidneys. The breakdown of fat, for its part, produces acetate and ketone bodies. Although some of the tissues in the body can use ketone bodies for fuel, they are not an ideal fuel for the body, and they are not a good fuel for the brain. The brain does not function well when fat is used exclusively for fuel. Finally, of course, while you're cutting back on carbohydrates, you're increasing your intake of fat and cholesterol, which are instrumental in the development of atherosclerosis.

Although a low-carbohydrate diet may help you lose weight, it is not ideal from a standpoint of general health. As a neurologist, I should also point out that it is not ideal for the brain. The ideal fuel for the brain is glucose. In fact, glucose is the only clean-burning fuel for the brain. The brain needs glucose, and carbohydrates are its major source. This includes carbohydrates that rapidly increase glucose levels—those high on the glycemic index—and those that cause more gradual increases. The glycemic index is a tool developed to determine how quickly carbohydrates affect blood glucose. The index can be found in many books and on many Web sites, including those dedicated to nutrition and diabetes. Foods high on the index rapidly increase the amount of glucose in the blood; foods low on the index work more slowly.

Some experts believe that you should limit your intake of foods high on the glycemic index to avoid insulin resistance and weight gain. I don't believe the index has much bearing on stroke or stroke risk. In fact, its impact on overall health may be very limited unless you are already overweight or are known to have a problem with insulin resistance.

My best advice is to eat a mixture of carbohydrates—both low and high on the index—and to make carbohydrates a mainstay of your diet.

Adopting carbohydrates as dietary staples also follows my other guiding dietary principle: to eat what we humans were designed to eat. Our bodies and metabolism are not made for eating meat and other high-fat animal foods. When we eat them, we develop diseases that can kill us, like atherosclerosis and cancer. This is not true of such carnivorous animals as dogs and cats. I think this is Mother Nature's way of telling us something.

Although humans have eaten meat, dairy products, and eggs for millennia, it has only been in the past hundred years or so that these foods have taken center stage on our plates. During that same period, the occurrence rates of numerous diseases have increased. Although some of these changes undoubtedly relate to the increase in our life expectancy, research indicates that many of these diseases—including atherosclerosis, ischemic heart disease, and some forms of cancer—are diet-related. Although dogs, cats, and other carnivores can eat large amounts of fat and not develop atherosclerosis, humans cannot. Neither can rabbits, who thrive on plant foods.

Our bodies are clearly designed to eat fruits, vegetables, and grains. These foods, which consist primarily of carbohydrates, offer a wealth of vitamins, minerals, and other beneficial nutrients. Studies indicate that people who eat large amounts of fruits and vegetables have lower rates of such diseases as ischemic heart disease and cancer. These findings have been linked largely to the unique combinations of nutrients these foods provide. To obtain the most nutrient value from these foods, we should eat them whole and in their most natural state. Refining and processing strips these plant foods of many of their nutrients.

I believe that if we listen hard to what Mother Nature is telling us and try to eat whole, natural foods that are good for overall health as well as the health of our brain and cerebrovascular system, we'll eat what we were meant to eat and be healthier as a result. Such a diet is also far healthier for our planet and the rest of its inhabitants.

MY DIETARY GUIDELINES

If you read regularly about health and health issues, you're probably familiar with the standard "healthy diet" advice offered by the U.S. government and many national health organizations. These sources generally recommend a diet that limits fat intake to 30 percent of total calories and dietary cholesterol intake to 300 milligrams per day. These figures are significantly lower than the typical American diet, in which approximately 40 percent of calories come from fat and dietary cholesterol intake averages 400 milligrams per day, but they do not go far enough in preventing such risk factors as atherosclerosis. Although America is a leader in many aspects of health, we clearly come up short when it comes to diet. What we consider low-fat in this country would be considered high-fat in most other countries. In order to eat the healthy diet we were meant to eat, we need to rethink our definition of "low-fat" and "low-cholesterol" and our dependence on animal foods. And we need to increase our intake of beneficial foods.

My diet calls for a more significant reduction in saturated fat and cholesterol than the standard diet recommended for vascular health, but it is not a deprivation diet. I have followed this plan myself for the past twelve of my forty-nine years and have refined it for my patients. Many of my patients have seen their blood pressure and cholesterol levels drop significantly, without medication.

Beth's total cholesterol was 240 mg/dL when she came to see me for carotid artery blockage and an unruptured intracranial aneurysm. I laid out the basics of my diet plan for her, and during the first year, she reduced her cholesterol level to 188 mg/dL. Despite her lowered cholesterol, her carotid artery blockage increased. Both of us knew she needed to do more.

Although she had adopted many of the basic principles of my diet plan, Beth had trouble giving up meat and eggs. She couldn't seem to go the extra step. I explained to her that even though many physicians recommend a total cholesterol level of 200 mg/dL, atherosclerosis can still progress at that level, as it had in her case. Because surgery to open up her carotid artery would increase the risk of her aneurysm rupturing, I told her she needed to do whatever she could with lifestyle to stop her carotid blockage from progressing.

Once she understood the gravity of her condition, she redoubled her efforts on the diet. The decisive factor—as it so often is when it comes to dietary changes—was a supportive spouse. After seeing films of her carotid blockage, her husband not only adopted a meatless and eggless diet, he took a special vegetarian cooking course to ensure that she'd have appetizing enough meals to stay on her diet. Six months later, her blockage had stabilized and her cholesterol was down to 150 mg/dL. Five years later, Beth is still stroke-free, with no progression of her carotid blockage.

Many of my patients have also lost a good deal of weight on this plan. (It has helped me keep my weight stable through middle age.) I can also attest that my patients report that after a few months on this diet, they simply feel better—less sluggish and healthier. I hope these broad benefits will motivate you to get on this plan, and stay on it. The plan works because it offers a pragmatic, sustainable approach to healthy eating. I've structured it so that the focus is on what you can eat, not simply what you can't eat.

The basic recipe for my plan is as follows:

> 10 to 20 percent of total daily calories from dietary fat in the
>   following ratio: 1 part saturated/trans to 3 parts
>   monounsaturated to 2 parts polyunsaturated.
> 10 to 20 percent of total daily calories from protein
> 60 to 70 percent of total daily calories from carbohydrates
> 10 milligrams or less of cholesterol per day
> 3,000 milligrams or less of sodium per day

If this is confusing to you, don't worry. I explain how this translates into what you can and should eat later in this chapter. First, let me offer an explanation. To prevent atherosclerosis from developing, I firmly believe that fat intake should be reduced to less than 20 percent of total calories and cholesterol intake should be reduced to 10 milligrams per day. Your body manufactures its own cholesterol—from the food you eat, primarily from saturated fat. If you consume high amounts of fat, particularly too much saturated fat, and/or high amounts of cholesterol, your total blood cholesterol level, as well as your level of low-density lipoprotein (LDL), will rise. LDL cholesterol is known as the "bad" cholesterol because excess amounts circulate in the bloodstream and can become incorporated into atherosclerotic deposits in artery walls.

This is why you need to watch your intake of saturated fat and cholesterol. Saturated fat, which comes from meat, dairy products, and eggs and is hard at room temperature, is the most unhealthy of the fats. It raises blood levels of LDL cholesterol. Trans fats, or trans fatty acids, which are found in products that contain hydrogenated vegetable oil, shortening, and margarine, act in a similar fashion. These fats, which may soon be listed on food labels, should be considered in the same category as saturated fat. Together with saturated fat, they should make up the smallest portion of your fat intake. Polyunsaturated fats, the predominant fat in such vegetable oils as corn, safflower, sunflower, and walnut, are of slightly less concern. They do not raise LDL cholesterol levels; however, they lower levels of high-density cholesterol (HDL). This "good" cholesterol helps escort LDL cholesterol to the liver and out of the body. The best of the fats are the monounsaturated fats. These fats, found in olive and canola oils, neither raise LDL cholesterol nor lower HDL cholesterol. And olive oil is also rich in vitamin E.

My diet plan calls for a saturated/trans to monounsaturated fat to polyunsaturated fat ratio of 1:3:2. If you get 18 percent of your daily calories from fat, this would translate into 3 percent saturated/trans fats, 9 percent monounsaturated fat, and 6 percent polyunsaturated fat. This means making olive and canola oil staples in your cooking. It means avoiding lard, butter, and vegetable oils with saturated fat like coconut and palm. It means using olive oil, pureed avocado, roasted garlic, jam, Benecol Spread or Take Control (butter substitutes that reduce LDL cholesterol) or mayonnaise substitutes like Vegenaise and Lite Canola Mayo in place of butter, regular margarine, or mayonnaise on your bread. Depending on what you eat now, it could also mean more substantial dietary changes.

To reduce your fat and cholesterol intake to the levels I recommend, you need to reduce—or, better yet, eliminate—your intake of animal foods, like meat, eggs, and dairy products—which are high in both saturated fat and cholesterol. This may sound extreme, but it doesn't necessarily mean depriving yourself or abandoning your favorite foods.

Numerous products on the market can help you give up meats without giving up any of their flavor or texture. Low-fat and nonfat dairy products and nondairy substitutes also abound. The number of products is growing steadily, and many are available in regular supermarkets as well as health food stores. In fact, the growing availability of such meat substitutes as meatless burgers, veggie hot dogs, meatless sausages, meatless bacon, chicken substitutes, and fish substitutes has had a major impact on the success of my patients. Many of them grew up on farms in the Midwest and were accustomed to eating meat and dairy products throughout the day. They have found that these alternative products can help them maintain the diet to which they are accustomed in terms of taste, smell, and texture while improving their health.

These products have also made eating a more enjoyable experience for me. When I first began following this eating plan twelve years ago, few meat substitutes were available, and many of the ones that were didn't really capture the flavor or texture of the meat to which I was accustomed. I grew up in Nebraska, the beef state. I was used to eating meat up to four times a day—at each meal and often as a bedtime snack. Although I never regretted changing my diet, for years I missed some of the tastes and flavors from my childhood. Now, I can have my "meat" and eat it, too. And BLTs—made with veggie bacon—have once again become a favorite snack.

I encourage you to experiment with the products available. They vary tremendously in taste. Although you might not like them all, you're bound to find something that appeals to you.

One of my patients, Walter, has meticulously followed the diet I recommend in this book for five years. During his first year on the diet, he told me that though it took him a little while, he had found some very good substitute meat and dairy products, but that he found a particular brand of sausage links and patties to be too peppery for him. I hadn't noticed. When I tried them again, I realized that he was right. They were peppery, which is why I like them, but that flavor ruled them out for him.

Veggie burgers are another good example of products that appeal to different tastes. Some mimic the taste of meat and resemble real hamburgers; others offer the unique taste of different blends of vegetables and grains. Dozens of these burgers are available in a whole range of styles and spices. You can eat one type one night and another type the next and not feel as if you've eaten the same thing two nights in a row. It can be a lot of fun to discover some of these new tastes and new flavors. You may find that you actually prefer certain products to meat. (Throughout this section, I'll be recommending meat substitutes. For the record, any brand recommendations I may make in this regard are strictly a matter of taste. I have never been paid to endorse any products.)

Meat Substitutes

Here are some of my favorite meat substitutes.

Bacon Substitutes

Morningstar Farms Breakfast Strips
Yves Veggie Canadian Bacon

Hamburger/Beef Substitutes

Lightlife Light Burgers

Gardenburger—hamburger style

Lightlife Smart Cutlets "Salisbury Steak"

Nate's Meatless Meatballs

Chicken Substitutes

VEAT breasts, kabobs, or chunks

Boca Meatless Nuggets

Turkey Substitutes

Tofurky Hickory Smoked Deli Slices

Tofurky Roast

Now & Zen Roast Vegetarian Turkey

Sausage Substitutes

H&Y Vienna Sausage Links

Morningstar Farms Breakfast Links

Lightlife Gimme Lean! Veggie Sausage

Hot Dog Substitutes

Yves Veggie Wieners

Natural Touch Vegetarian Franks

Morningstar Farms Veggie Dogs

If you absolutely must eat meat, make fish your choice. Although fish are subject to water contamination and pollution, and farm-raised fish are routinely given antibiotics and, because of their diet, are generally not as rich in vital nutrients, fish do offer protein and omega-3 fatty acids, which may offer health benefits. You may also obtain omega-3 fatty acids from free-range eggs. These acids are available in supplement form, and plenty of tasty fish substitutes—as well as egg substitutes—are available. Chicken and turkey offer only minor advantages over red meat and are best avoided.

My eating plan focuses on such wholesome, fresh foods as fruits and vegetables, as well as grains, nonfat dairy products, and meat substitutes. These are the ingredients of a healthy diet. They are rich in vitamins, minerals, and other nutrients, rich in fiber and low in fat, cholesterol, and sodium. Although we tend to equate sodium with salt, we're more likely to get this mineral from processed and prepared foods than from our salt shakers. Eating fresh foods—particularly whole foods—can help reduce sodium intake as well as preserve naturally occurring nutrients that may be lost during food preparation.

Sodium can be a problem, particularly if you have a family history of hypertension or are known to be sodium sensitive. Sodium is known to raise blood pressure in sodium-sensitive individuals. Although there is some disagreement about whether a widespread reduction in sodium intake would result in fewer people developing hypertension, a reduction can affect your individual tendency to develop hypertension if you are sodium sensitive. Since most people do not know if they are sodium sensitive—and because the American diet is very high in sodium—I recommend that you limit your sodium intake to less than 3,000 milligrams a day.

This doesn't mean you have to throw away your salt shaker; it simply means that you have to use it judiciously and pay attention to the sodium content of the prepared foods you eat. The amount is listed on the Nutrition Facts label. If you don't make a habit of reading food labels, you may be unpleasantly surprised to find how many "nonsalty" foods are high in sodium. On the flip side, if you cut down on your use of salt while cooking, you may be pleasantly surprised to see what flavors you've been missing.

I list the basic foods you can eat on my plan below. They can be combined and prepared in numerous ways, offering you a lifetime of tasty, healthy meals. For suggestions on how to make the most of these ingredients, I include some of my favorite cookbooks in the suggested reading section at the back of the book.

Foods You Can Eat

One of the primary reasons my patients have success with my diet plan is that I focus on what they *can* eat, rather than what they can't. I don't simply give them a list of forbidden foods and say, "Follow this diet." Instead, I provide them with a list of foods they can eat. This list is broken down into foods they can eat anytime and foods they can eat sometimes. They can eat as much as they want of the "anytime" foods, which, in many cases, means they can actually eat *more* food on this plan if they so choose.

Here is the list I provide to my patients.

ANYTIME

Fruits and Vegetables	Fruits and Vegetables (cont'd)	Dairy	Beans, Eggs, Meat Substitutes
Fresh, frozen, canned, dried, or juiced: Apples, apricots, bananas, blackberries, blueberries, cantaloupe, cherries, cranberries, currants, dates, figs, gooseberries, grapefruit, grapes, honeydew, kiwis, lemons, limes, mangoes, mulberries, nectarines, oranges, peaches, pears, pineapples, plums, pomegranates, prunes, raisins, raspberries, star fruits, strawberries, tangerines, watermelon, fruit ices, sorbets *Fresh, frozen, canned, dried, or juiced:* Artichokes, asparagus, beans (green, wax, lima) beets, broccoli, brussels sprouts, cabbage, carrots, cauliflower, celery, collards, corn, cucumbers, dandelion greens, eggplant, escarole, fennel, garlic, kale, kelp, leeks, lentils, lettuce, mushrooms (button, cup, flat, chanterelle, morel,	oyster, shiitake, etc.), mustard greens, okra, onions, parsnips, peas, peppers (bell, chile), potatoes (baked, mashed), radishes, rutabagas, snow peas, spinach, sprouts (alfalfa, mustard, bean, radish), squash, sweet potato (baked, mashed), Swiss chard, tomato, turnips, turnip greens **Grains** Whole-grain breads, bagels, breadsticks, English muffins, pita bread, plain rolls, hot and cold whole-grain cereals (corn, oats, rye, wheat, barley, bulgur, millet, quinoa, buckwheat), rice (brown, white, wild), grits, macaroni, pasta, non-egg noodles, corn tortillas, air-popped popcorn, pretzels, fat-free crackers, fat-free cookies, fat-free muffins	Fat-free nondairy desserts, nonfat soy milk, nonfat rice milk, soy shakes, fat-free cheese substitutes **Fats** Fat-free chocolate, fat-free salad dressing, fat-free non-dairy creamer **Miscellaneous** Fat-free vegetarian chili and other soups (split pea, lentil, vegetable)	Beans (kidney, garbanzo, pinto, black, brown, white, great northern, mung, navy, red, Mexican, lima), lentils, peas (split, black-eyed), soybean products (tofu, tempeh, miso), Seitan (wheat gluten), egg whites, fat-free meat substitutes,* including veggie burgers, veggie hot dogs, veggie Canadian bacon, veggie chicken, veggie turkey with or without vegetarian gravy, and veggie breakfast strips, links, and patties

* As long as it contains no saturated fat or cholesterol

SOMETIMES

Fruits and Vegetables	Grains	Dairy	Beans, Eggs, Meat Substitutes
Avocado, coconut, olives, vegetables in low-fat cheese sauce,* vegetables in low-fat cream sauce*	Very-low-fat snack foods, low-fat snack foods (low-fat popcorn, low-fat chips, crackers, cake),* egg noodles **Fats** Low-fat salad dressing, olive oil and other vegetable oils with little saturated fat and no cholesterol	Skim milk, nonfat yogurt, fat-free sour cream, fat-free cream cheese, fat-free cottage cheese, low-fat yogurt,* low-fat sour cream,* low-fat cream cheese,* low-fat cottage cheese,* low-fat cheese* **Miscellaneous** Vegetarian pot pie with meat substitute, low-fat vegetarian enchiladas, low-fat vegetarian burritos, roasted vegetable pizza with vegetarian or low-fat cheese topping	Nuts (peanuts walnuts, pecans, almonds, Brazil nuts, etc.), seeds (sesame, pumpkin, sunflower, etc.) egg substitute, textured vegetable protein,* veggie burgers,* meatless breakfast strips,* links and patties,* meatless ground beef substitutes,* meatless chicken breast,* patties,* kebabs,* meatless Buffalo wings, meatless Salisbury steak,* meatless cocktail wieners,* meatless fish fillet,* meatless salmon steaks,* lentil loaf*

As long as they are less than 7 grams of total fat and less than 2 grams of saturated fat per serving

AVOID

Fruits and Vegetables	Grains	Dairy	Meats, Eggs
Fried vegetables, vegetables in regular cheese, cream sauce, or butter, vegetables in margarine	Regular cake, regular chips, chow mein noodles, regular cookies, regular crackers, croissants, doughnuts, granola, regular muffins, pies, regular popcorn, regular snack foods, stuffing, sweet rolls	Whole or 2 percent milk, whole or reduced-fat yogurt, reduced-fat or regular cheese, ice cream, cream, reduced fat or regular sour cream, reduced fat or regular cream cheese, reduced fat or regular cottage cheese	Meats (including poultry, fish, and seafood), egg yolks

Fats

Most margarines, regular salad dressings, oils with large amounts of saturated fat (coconut, palm, palm kernel, etc.), butter, lard, shortening, regular nondairy creamers, regular or milk chocolate

Foods to Avoid

Although I believe the list of foods you can eat is of more benefit than a list of foods you should avoid, I include the latter for your reference. If you compare the two lists, you will see that the list of foods you can eat contains many substitutes for foods on this list.

Foods and Nutrients That Offer Special Benefits

Following my general dietary guidelines will give you a firm foundation of healthy eating and a lot of beneficial nutrients, particularly if you focus on fresh fruits and vegetables. But you can—and should—take steps to get even more out of your food. Preliminary evidence suggests that certain foods may offer additional, independent protection against stroke. This may be due, in part, to the nutrients they contain. Vitamins and minerals may do more than simply keep us from developing deficiency diseases— they may protect us against other types of diseases as well. To maintain optimum health, I believe we must ensure that we get adequate amounts of nutrients known to be essential—from foods and supplements. And we need to take specific advantage of foods that may offer health benefits independent of vitamins and minerals. After all, many components of food have not yet been isolated and researched.

Foods You Should Eat

For years, studies have linked high fruit and vegetable intake to better overall health, including a reduced risk of cancer and heart disease. Some studies have also linked fruit and vegetable intake to a reduced risk of stroke, although the connection was not firmly established. In 1999, researchers from the Harvard School of Public Health offered the strongest data to date on the matter. After monitoring the health and diets of 75,596 women and 38,683 men for fourteen and eight years, respectively, they found that those who ate five to six servings of fruits and vegetables a day were 31 percent less likely to have an ischemic stroke than those who ate fewer than three servings. Each daily serving was associated with a 6 percent reduction in risk. The most potent effects were found in orange juice and other citrus fruits and juices, green leafy vegetables, and such cruciferous vegetables as broccoli, cabbage, brussels sprouts, and cauliflower. Needless to say, these are all on the list of foods you can eat. I also put them on a new list: a list of foods you *should* eat.

Another food to add to that list is soy. This protein, derived from soybeans, is perhaps the most ideal form of protein available. It's inexpensive, low in fat, and research indicates that it may actually lower your blood LDL cholesterol levels. Several studies have found that people who regularly substitute soy for animal protein can reduce their total cholesterol levels by up to 10 percent. Other research indicates that soy may protect against cancer, osteoporosis, and hot flashes during menopause, although this evidence is less conclusive. To obtain optimal cholesterol-lowering benefits from soy, you need to eat at least 25 grams of soy protein a day. Good sources include soy milk, tofu, tempeh, and textured vegetable protein, which is found in many meat substitutes.

You should also try to get omega-3 fatty acids, which may reduce blood levels of triglycerides, make blood less likely to clot, and dampen the inflammatory response. These fatty acids have been linked to a reduced risk of ischemic heart disease. Most people know that omega-3 fatty acids are found in cold-water fish. As I noted earlier, they may also be found in the yolks of free-range chicken eggs, largely because these chickens eat a variety of vegetable sources, and in supplements. Omega-3 fatty acids are also found in vegetable sources, including flaxseed and flaxseed oil, soybeans and soybean oil, walnuts and walnut oil, seaweed, and an edible plant known as purslane. At the same time, you should reduce intake of omega-6 fatty acids, which, though essential, are too prevalent in the typical American diet. If intake of these fats, found in meat, poultry, and corn, cottonseed, grapeseed, peanut, safflower, sesame, soybean, and sunflower oils, far exceeds intake of omega-3 fatty acids, the body may not produce hormones known as inhibitory prostaglandins, which protect the body from various diseases and conditions.

Supplements

Clearly, fruits and vegetables offer a wealth of beneficial nutrients. If you eat plenty of fruits and vegetables and follow my general dietary advice, you will reach the recommended dietary allowances of most essential vitamins and minerals. In fact, my diet should be the primary means by which you meet these goals. As I've said, foods, particularly whole, natural foods, contain many components, including some we have not identified and isolated. Still, to ensure that you are getting adequate amounts of all the known essential vitamins and minerals, I recommend that you take a daily multivitamin-mineral supplement.

Your own personal taste and selection, the way you prepare your food, and its freshness—or lack thereof—can all affect the nutrient content of your overall diet. Certain nutrients, like vitamin E, which is found primarily in high-fat foods, are hard to come by in a low-fat diet. For optimal health, we need more of certain nutrients than the recommended dietary allowances. These guidelines, which are currently being overhauled, were originally designed to reflect the minimum amounts of nutrients needed for health. This is why I advocate a daily multivitamin-mineral supplement.

Not all multivitamin-mineral supplements provide the amounts I believe are needed for health, so additional supplements may also be warranted, particularly of the antioxidants—vitamins C and E, selenium, and beta carotene. These nutrients, which neutralize potentially dangerous oxidative reactions in the body, have been ascribed with healing powers that rival any miracle drug. Although many of these claims have not yet been proven, I do believe antioxidants have some value, and I don't believe they are harmful when they are consumed in reasonable doses.

Because the content of different multivitamin-mineral supplements varies, and you may be able to find some products that offer the amounts you need of certain nutrients but not of others, I provide you with my recommendations for what I believe you should take in each day. You may need to add supplements of individual nutrients to your multi to achieve these amounts.

Vitamin A in the form of mixed carotenoids, including 20,000 to
   30,000 International Units of beta carotene

Vitamin B_1 (thiamin)	10 milligrams
Vitamin B_2 (riboflavin)	10 milligrams
Vitamin B_3 (niacin)	100 milligrams
Vitamin B_6	10 milligrams
Vitamin B_{12}	50 micrograms
Folate	400 micrograms
Vitamin C	200 milligrams
Vitamin D	400–800 International Units

Vitamin E	400–800 International Units
Calcium	1,500 milligrams
Selenium	100–200 micrograms
Iron	18–36 milligrams (in divided doses, if necessary)

ALCOHOL AND CAFFEINE

Two other "food groups" warrant some discussion: alcohol and caffeine. I won't tell you to give up either completely; in fact, some people may benefit from an occasional toast "to your health." But I do want to offer some guidance on these popular drugs.

Alcohol

As I explain in chapter 2, alcohol is a mixed bag when it comes to stroke. Light to moderate drinking appears to have a beneficial effect in preventing atherosclerotic ischemic stroke, but drinking also appears to increase the risk of hemorrhagic stroke, particularly heavy drinking and binge drinking, which are unhealthy for a number of reasons.

If you have risk factors for atherosclerotic stroke—say, you have a family history of atherosclerosis or you've long eaten a high-fat, high-cholesterol diet—you may benefit from having an occasional drink, but no more than two per day. If, on the other hand, you have any risk factors for hemorrhagic stroke, for example, a family history of intracranial aneurysms or hypertension, you may wish to avoid alcohol altogether.

Caffeine

Caffeine is our culture's most commonly used "upper." It's in our coffee, our soft drinks, even our chocolate. Along with giving us a slight buzz, it causes a temporary increase in our blood pressure. This is of little concern to most people, but could provide a slightly increased risk to someone with an unruptured intracranial aneurysm or an arteriovenous malformation, especially if it is consumed several cups at a time. Although all the information is not in, temporary spikes in blood pressure may cause aneurysms and vascular malformations to rupture, causing hemorrhagic stroke. If you're prone to either of these conditions—perhaps you have a family history of intracranial aneurysms or you have one of the conditions that are linked to aneurysm development—you may wish to cut back on your morning coffee or drink decaf.

PUTTING IT ALL TOGETHER

To help you put all the various aspects of the Stroke-Free for Life diet into action, I provide you with several sample menu plans designed to show you what you can and should eat. (See chart on page 206.)

Exercise

I love to extol exercise. I can't think of any activity more healthful. No doubt you know that exercise tones and strengthens your muscles and helps you maintain your body weight or contributes to weight loss. You also know that it increases your endurance, flexibility, and energy level. Did you know that it eases the pain and stiffness of arthritis, strengthens bones and protects them against osteoporosis, improves your mood, and may reduce the risk of certain forms of cancer? More important for our purposes, did you know that exercise helps reduce the risk of numerous stroke risk factors? Regular exercise improves the health of the heart and blood vessels, reduces blood pressure, increases the level of high-density lipoprotein (HDL), the so-called good cholesterol, in the blood, prevents or helps control diabetes mellitus, reduces stress, and counteracts some of the symptoms of depression. Regular exercise has also been shown in several recent studies actually to reduce the risk of stroke. And exercise releases chemicals known as endorphins that make us feel good.

Needless to say, regular exercise is a powerful stroke preventive. It attacks stroke on many fronts, preventing or controlling various conditions that increase risk. And it offers other health benefits as well. There's only one drawback to this prescription for prevention: just as many drugs must be taken regularly and in a certain amount, exercise must be performed regularly for a certain amount of time to offer its full benefits. An infrequent workout isn't going to do you much good and, in fact, may do you harm.

THE EXERCISE PRESCRIPTION

The good news about this exercise prescription is that it isn't a hard pill to swallow. You don't need to go to the pharmacy to fill it, although you should check with your doctor before starting to find out if you have any

Sample Meal Plans*

	Day 1	Day 2	Day 3	Day 4	Day 5	Day 6	Day 7
BREAKFAST	banana bread (fat free) with Benecol or Take Control (spread) blueberries oatmeal soy milk or skim milk	buckwheat pancakes strawberries—fresh or sauce pineapple juice	cereal (whole grain, fat free) raisins or banana whole wheat toast with Benecol or Take Control soy milk or skim milk orange juice	bagel marmalade or all-fruit jam peanut butter or almond butter red and green grapes	egg substitute omelet w/veggies salsa topping fresh grapefruit or juice English muffin with Benecol, Take Control, or all-fruit jam	muffin (fat free) yogurt (fat free) peach slices or juice	melon and kiwi cottage cheese (fat free) cinnamon toast with Benecol or Take Control apple juice
LUNCH	bean taco with lettuce/tomato salsa/fat-free sour cream or plain yogurt mixed vegetable salad with cherry tomatoes fat-free salad dressing plum and orange slices	spicy black bean veggie burger hamburger bun (whole grain) catsup/mustard tomato/lettuce/onion watermelon salad steamed vegetables	bacon, lettuce, and tomato sandwich made with meatless bacon substitute split pea soup* peach	pasta with tomato sauce with cooked veggies (broccoli, carrots, cauliflower, mushrooms, spinach, peppers) and ground beef substitute from textured vegetable protein bread sticks (fat free) apple slices	vegetable soup* crackers (whole grain) orange slices raw vegetables (carrots, bell peppers, pea pods)	baked potato with fat-free bean chili mixed lettuce salad with fat-free salad dressing cherries	peanut butter or almond butter whole-grain bread all-fruit jam banana, pineapple, melon oatmeal cookie (fat free)
EVENING	vegetarian shepherd's pie* cucumber salad with yogurt dressing sorbet topped with raspberries	oven roasted vegetables with pasta* crusty Italian bread with Benecol or Take Control fresh mixed fruit	green bean dinner medley* Oriental green salad orange fruit ice with blackberries	lentil loaf mashed potatoes with fresh tomato sauce* or noodles with wild mushroom gravy* green salad cantaloupe and honeydew	portobello mushroom burgers* soy or low-fat cheese sliced red onion whole-grain bun carrot salad mixed fruit over cake (fat free)	bell peppers stuffed with Spanish rice* cornbread (fat free) green salad pear salad with maraschino cherry	potatoes risotto* asparagus and red peppers with lemon juice spinach salad with toasted almonds applesauce spice cake (fat free)

limitations and what your exercise parameters should be. You don't need to run the marathon or overwork yourself to benefit, although generally you need to get a little bit winded. Even such moderate exercise as brisk walking will do the trick. You don't need to give up hours of your time or diligently watch a clock to make sure you're timing your dosage correctly. You can even split up your dosage, "taking" a little at one time and a little at another. All you need to do is make sure you get at least thirty minutes of aerobic exercise at least three times a week. You're welcome to get more, of course. It's hard to overdose on exercise.

You can overdo it, though, and you can hurt yourself. To make sure that you don't, warm up before you exercise and monitor your heart rate during aerobic exercise. Aerobic exercise is exercise that increases the body's demand for oxygen, including walking, running, and swimming. It involves continuous, rhythmic contracting of large muscles, increases the rate and depth of breathing, increases heart rate, and is the best type of exercise for reducing stroke risk. To ensure that you are working out at the proper intensity, you want your heart rate to be between 50 and 80 percent of its maximal exercise capacity. You can figure out your maximal heart rate by subtracting your age from the number 220. If you are fifty, your maximal heart rate is 170. Your target heart rate is 50 to 80 percent of that number, or 85 to 136 beats per minute.

You can determine your heart rate by taking your pulse during your workout. Stop exercising and place two fingers on the thumb side of your wrist, between the bone and tendon, to feel the pulsing of your radial artery. Count the number of pulse beats for ten seconds, then multiply by six to determine the number of beats per minute.

YOUR EXERCISE OPTIONS

Okay, so you know how often and how intensely you should exercise, but what can you do? That's the other good thing about this prescription— you have a choice. Many types of exercise are available, and you can—and should—choose an activity or activities that you enjoy. If you do, you'll be much more likely to stick to your exercise program. Your program doesn't have to be formal or limited. You can alternate a variety of activities and exercises that appeal to you, perhaps swimming one day and walking or working in your garden on another. Variety is, after all, the spice of life. And it can keep you from getting bored with your exercise routine.

As I said, the best type of exercise for stroke prevention is aerobic exercise. Many people equate this with running or jogging, but it doesn't have to be that intense. Walking at a brisk pace can produce similar aerobic effects, so can swimming, dancing, tennis, racquetball, bicycling, cross-country skiing, golf (if you walk briskly and carry or pull your clubs), hiking and mountain climbing (two of my favorites), and formal aerobics classes.

You're bound to find an activity that works for you. If you have a bad back, try swimming or bicycling. If you have arthritis, you might find swimming soothing. If you like to exercise alone, consider walking or bicycling. If you like to exercise with others, consider taking a class or finding a tennis partner. If you have a large house and yard, you have an incentive to include household chores and gardening among your options.

Isometric exercise is generally less beneficial with more opportunity for harm than aerobic exercise, although lifting small amounts of weight at high repetitions can have aerobic benefits. Isometric exercises isolate muscles and cause rapid, short-term increases in blood pressure. As I mentioned above, these spikes can theoretically increase your risk of hemorrhage if you have an unruptured intracranial aneurysm or vascular malformation.

Stress Reduction

The final lifestyle component of the Stroke-Free for Life Plan is stress reduction. Like exercise—which, incidentally, is a great way to blow off steam—stress reduction benefits the entire body and makes you feel good. I believe it also reduces the risk of stroke.

Our bodies respond to stress by releasing the stress hormones cortisol and epinephrine (adrenaline) into the system. These hormones cause the heart to beat faster, blood pressure to rise, muscles to tense, and senses to sharpen. These reactions essentially prepare the body to react to immediate physical danger. In fact, that's what they are designed to do. The stress response is also known as the "fight-or-flight" response, and it has helped humans survive numerous physical dangers over the millennia.

Unfortunately, we can't fight or flee many of the "dangers" we face in today's society. Our bodies don't entirely recognize the difference between physical danger and other causes of worry, overwork, illness, and internal conflicts, for example. Yet these stressors are increasingly common. What's more, many of them don't go away quickly. As a result, our autonomic nervous system continues to release these hormones into our bodies, with unhealthy effects. Stress hormones increase both heart rate and blood pressure. In addition, cortisol has been found to raise blood cholesterol levels and accelerate the development of atherosclerosis.

Although few studies have actually focused on stress as a risk factor for stroke, it has been implicated as a risk factor for ischemic heart disease and also for depression (both risk factors for ischemic stroke), and there is reason to believe that the cardiovascular changes caused by stress hormones can affect stroke risk.

Even if stress does not turn out to be a strong, independent risk factor for stroke, it is likely to have some effect on stroke risk. You can't go wrong by reducing stress. Research indicates that reducing stress can improve overall health and well-being. The best way to do this, in my opinion, is by making lifestyle changes. Although medications are available to reduce stress, they should be used only for the short term. Lifestyle changes are the best long-term methods of stress reduction—and they can be remarkably successful, especially if you choose ones that apply to your individual situation and appeal to your taste.

Jeffrey was a forty-five-year-old futures trader in the Chicago commodities exchange. Every day was stressful for him, with hundreds of thousands of dollars hanging in the balance as he bought and sold futures contracts on soybeans, sugar, and wheat. He spent six hours a day shouting and gesturing in a crowded "pit," then unwound by drinking every late afternoon before he went home. Even in my exam room, Jeff was in constant motion. When he came to see me, he was suffering from hypertension, coronary artery disease, chest pains, and TIA-like spells. He was clearly worried about his health, but initially he insisted that there was nothing he could do about his work-related stress. He was hoping I could prescribe medication.

I knew that medication would help him cope only in the short term. Instead, I took a thorough history, looked at his diet, and talked to him about what else was going on in his life. It turned out that his work wasn't his only source of stress. His marriage had been deteriorating for some years, and he had responded by pouring more of himself into his work. (Not surprisingly, many of his marital problems stemmed from the fact that he was always so stressed out from work.) Even though he made a lot of money, it was all on commissions, so he worried it could go away overnight and leave him with nothing but a big mortgage and private school tuitions.

I'm not a psychotherapist, but it was obvious to me that Jeff had to reexamine his priorities if he hoped to survive into his fifties. I told him what I saw down the road for him, and it wasn't a pretty picture. He said he was serious about making some changes in his life. We dealt with the simple things first. We cut his caffeine intake from ten cups a day to two. Within a week, he realized that more stimulus was the last thing he needed, so he cut out the last two cups himself. Instead of eating lunch on his feet, often while still trading, I convinced him to bring a healthy meal to work and find a quiet office to eat in. Instead of controlling his stress with alcohol, I convinced him to find an after-work meditation group. As it happened, there was a group of traders who met at a gym around the corner and did a combination of yoga and breathing meditation.

Once he started to slow down a bit, something interesting happened. A few weeks later, Jeff confided to me that he wasn't enjoying the trading as much anymore. It just felt like an addiction—or at least a compulsion. "You know, I used to love the pit. It's where the action was, where I wanted to be." He shook his head and smiled a little sadly. "Now all I see is a bunch of guys jumping up and down and shouting at each other. Maybe I'm just too old for it." A few months later, Jeff was able to get a job managing other traders. It was a lot calmer than life "in the pit," the pay was steadier, and he actually enjoyed it more. Most important, his health improved. His chest pains went away, his hypertension faded, and he stopped having fainting spells.

Sometimes, illness itself can be a dangerous stressor. Barbara is a perfect example. The fifty-year-old high school teacher came to see me after she was diagnosed with a small unruptured intracranial aneurysm. She initially saw a neurosurgeon who advised her to have the aneurysm surgically clipped immediately. Paralyzed with fear, she went straight to the hospital while her husband went back home to get her things. By the time she arrived at the hospital, she was thinking a little more clearly and decided to get a second opinion. Neurosurgeons and endovascular neuroradiologists at two local academic medical centers told her that the operation might not be necessary. By that time, she was so stricken with fear and confusion that she had been unable to function for about a month. That's when she came to see me.

In a one-hour phone discussion and two subsequent discussions in person, I explained to her that the International Study of Unruptured Intracranial Aneurysms indicated that the likelihood that her aneurysm would rupture was about $\frac{1}{20}$ of 1 percent per year, which means that it would take approximately twenty years for her to reach a 1 percent chance of rupture. I also explained that the surgical procedure to treat the aneurysm carried a death and disability rate of around 10 percent. I reassured her that she could lead a normal lifestyle. Normally an exerciser, she had stopped exercising after her diagnosis because she had been afraid it would cause her aneurysm to rupture. This, in turn, had heightened her stress level. With the reassurance and the exercise and relaxation techniques described in this book, she was able to conquer her fear, control her stress, and resume her normal lifestyle.

Needless to say, there are numerous ways to reduce stress, from physically addressing the fight-or-flight response with exercise (another major component of the Stroke-Free for Life Plan), to reducing the number of stressors in your life, from finding outlets to deflect stress to trying a relaxation technique.

REDUCING STRESSORS

One of the best ways to reduce your stress level is to eliminate your stressors—the things that cause you stress. This approach gets to the root of the problem, although it cannot be used with every stressor. If you know what aspects of your life are causing you stress, and you have control over them, you can take steps to reduce their impact. If you're overwhelmed by responsibilities, for example, you may be able to cut back on some of your activities or better organize yourself to cope with your duties. You can also take a tip from drug abuse prevention efforts and "just say no" when someone asks you to add another responsibility to your list. Make lists of your goals and duties; prioritize your duties; delegate some of your responsibilities to others, if possible; make good use of your time; and don't put things off—it only makes matters worse.

Following these suggestions can help you even if your major stressors are beyond your control. There is no way to avoid dealing with the illness or death of a loved one, for example, but taking steps to eliminate the other, smaller stressors in your life when you are dealing with such major problems can reduce your overall stress level.

The Causes and Symptoms of Stress

Stress has numerous causes and manifests itself in numerous ways. We all face difficult situations, and we all react differently. For example, although one person may become more focused as a deadline approaches, another may have difficulty concentrating, become irritable, or actually become physically ill. Symptoms of stress range from restlessness, impatience, and obsessive working, to fatigue, insomnia, and loss of concentration, as well as a host of physical symptoms, from nausea and vomiting to rashes, headaches, sweaty palms, and tight muscles. Stress has been linked to such illnesses as depression, ulcers, and ischemic heart disease. Research indicates it lowers our resistance to illness and makes us more susceptible to colds and flu.

The triggers for these reactions range from such major life events as a death, birth, marriage, and divorce, to everyday dealings with our jobs and families. Stressors are not necessarily negative. Positive events like marriage, job promotions, and even vacations can trigger stress. Just about anything can cause stress on a given day, depending on your mood and the other stresses in your life. As a result, no definitive list of stressors can be compiled. What follows is a list of some of the many stressors that have been identified. Use it as a guide to help you determine what situations or events in your own life are causing you stress.

Aging
Birth of a child
Change in eating habits
Change in exercise habits
Death of a friend or loved one
Financial difficulties

Holidays

Illness or injury (personal or of a friend or loved one)

Job difficulties (role ambiguity, work overload, not getting along with your boss or coworkers, being promoted, being demoted, changing positions, being fired, etc.)

Moving

Retirement

Relationship difficulties with family or friends

FIND AN OUTLET

Another proven way to reduce stress is to find outlets to relieve your stress and take your mind off the things that are stressing you. Exercise is perfect for this. It answers the body's physical fight-or-flight need, focuses your attention on something else, and floods your body with endorphins that make you feel good emotionally. As I explain above, exercise has numerous other physical benefits for your body.

Exercise is not the only outlet available to you. Anytime you do something for yourself—spend time with a friend, read a good book, see a good movie, spend time on a hobby—you direct your attention away from what's stressing you to something more pleasant and relaxing. Relaxation is exactly what you need to counter the effects of stress. Here are some outlets I find particularly effective at reducing stress:

Laugh

In many cases, laughter *is* the best medicine. Research indicates that laughing increases blood flow to the brain, releases endorphins, and decreases levels of stress hormones. It relieves tension and apprehension and increases our ability to think positively. This, in turn, can lead to lower blood pressure and an increase in white blood cell production, which increases immunity. The benefits of laughter are being used in medicine, although not as widely as they might be. Some doctors schedule an hour of "laugh therapy" for their cancer patients on a daily basis. They see real benefit to this therapy, and much of that benefit comes from stress reduction. So let yourself laugh. Look for humor around you. See a funny movie. Read a humor column or a funny book. Visit a comedy club.

Find an Inspirational Place

We have all been somewhere where we felt at peace—a beach, a forest, a mountaintop. Spending some quiet time in a peaceful, inspiring place can help you tune in to yourself and focus on things other than the daily problems that are the root of your stress. It can also help you relax. If you have a favorite place, make a point to visit it. If you don't have a favorite place, find one. Visit a local park, take a walk in the woods, visit the nearest beach. Take some time for yourself.

Spend Time with a Companion Animal

Snoopy used to say, "Happiness is a warm puppy." Of course, the cartoon dog was biased, but he's not that far off. Many of us find it comforting to be around animals. Research has shown that interacting with a companion animal can lower blood pressure and heart rate and reduce anxiety. It can also improve mood. "Pet therapy," regular visits from companion animals, is a standard activity in many nursing homes and hospitals. At Mayo Clinic, some years ago, we changed our policy to allow companion animals to visit their human companions when they are ill. Research has shown that people who live with animals often heal faster and have better overall outcomes when they are ill than people who do not live with animals. This may be due to the strong emotional bond they have with the animal. Many people consider their companion animals family. In some cases, the animals are the only family members they have. Companion animals can help alleviate loneliness and give us someone to take care of.

Do Something for Someone Else

The single best thing you can do to help relieve your stress, in my opinion, is to focus attention on helping others. Empathy redirects your attention, reduces tension, and reduces the tendency to worry about yourself. Helping others can give you a deep personal fulfillment, redefine your sense of purpose and priorities, and engender joy and peace that can redirect and overcome stress. Volunteer at your local soup kitchen or animal shelter. Visit a friend—or a stranger—at your local hospital. Offer to run errands for your elderly neighbor. Set aside some time to talk with a friend who is facing a major decision or undergoing a life crisis.

Relaxation Techniques

True relaxation is more than just sitting down for a moment between errands. It slows and deepens your breathing, slows your heart rate, loosens your muscles, and clears your mind. In short, it physically counters the effects of stress. A variety of techniques can help you reach this state, although it takes skill and practice to master them. You can try them on your own or seek guidance. Many health centers, community colleges, and organizations like the YMCA and YWCA offer classes in certain relaxation techniques. The Self-Help and New Age sections of many bookstores are bursting at the shelves with books that detail relaxation strategies. I outline the basics of some of the major ones below, but I urge you to take the next step. Read more about those that interest you. Learn about others. Experiment with several and find one—or more—that you believe will work for you. Your intuition will be an important guide to you in this endeavor.

DEEP BREATHING

This technique is exactly what its name implies: a slow, controlled, rhythmic form of breathing that allows you to focus on relaxation rather than stress. To perform this technique, you stand or sit up straight; inhale slowly, letting your abdomen and ribs expand; then you exhale, first from the abdomen and then from the chest. Your concentration should be solely on your breathing.

Deep, rhythmic breathing can be performed on its own or as part of another relaxation technique. Breathing is central to *pranayama,* the yoga of breathing. It also plays a role in progressive muscle relaxation and many forms of visualization.

PROGRESSIVE MUSCLE RELAXATION

This technique teaches you to recognize physical stress in the form of tense muscles. It involves systematically contracting and relaxing individual muscles. To perform it, you stand or sit up straight, close your eyes, and begin deep breathing. Then, you begin to tense and relax each muscle in order from top to bottom (your toes to your head). Tapes are available to direct and guide you through the process, or you can make your own using a script you buy at a bookstore.

VISUALIZATION AND AFFIRMATION

This technique helps you fight stress by changing your perception of it or by focusing on a pleasant situation. Two techniques exist. In the first, you close your eyes and envision overcoming something that is causing you stress. You might, for example, visualize your stressor as purple circles that you can stuff into a garbage can and throw away. You could couple this by making an affirming statement, such as "I deal with stress easily and effortlessly." In the second technique, you close your eyes and imagine a pleasant scene or event or relive a pleasant memory. This type of visualization can be simple or complex, prepared or unprepared. You can be guided by prerecorded tapes or create one yourself. Or you can simply sit down and let your imagination run.

MEDITATION

This relaxation technique, which should be performed regularly, is designed to remove your consciousness temporarily from the stresses of life. Several varieties of meditation exist, but the hallmark of each is concentration on a single object and ignoring everything else. You sit or lie in a comfortable position and breathe deeply and rhythmically, then you silently and continuously repeat a word, concentrate on an object, your breath, or a lighted candle for example, or visualize an object to prevent being distracted.

YOGA

This ancient relaxation technique combines exercise and meditation. This Indian art, which was originally designed to achieve spiritual perfection, a union of the soul with God, encourages a balanced development of human potential. Many forms of yoga exist. The most popular in the United States is hatha yoga, which incorporates postures, regular breathing, and meditation and has been found to relieve stress and lower blood pressure.

Other forms of yoga include raja yoga, which focuses primarily on meditation and is designed to quiet the mind; mantra yoga, which focuses on the power of the word; bhakti yoga, which focuses on love and devotion; kundalini yoga, which focuses on heightening awareness and tapping inner energy; and karma yoga, which focuses on service. Various schools or paths of yoga incorporate different types of yoga. Yoga is often best learned by taking a class. You can also rent videotapes, or take them out from the library, if you're curious about trying different methods.

TAI CHI

Another ancient form of meditative exercise, tai chi involves slow, flowing body movements. It uses the body's full range of motion and helps promote physical strength as well as mental clarity and relaxation. Like yoga, many find it is best learned by taking a class.

MASSAGE

No doubt you know that a good back rub can make you feel more relaxed, both physically and mentally. Massage makes muscles loose, which helps you relax and counters the tension of stress. You can learn self-massage from a book or class or visit a trained masseur or masseuse who will massage your body for you. You can also have a masseur or physical therapist teach your significant other the techniques. This can make massage more accessible and more enjoyable.

SOUND

Exposing yourself to sounds, especially natural sounds, is another tried and true relaxation technique. Sound waves have a direct effect on the brain— an effect that can be quite relaxing. Just think of some of the sounds you enjoy: music, birds, crickets, the sound of waves crashing against the shore. Sound also plays a role in other relaxation techniques. A mantra, or chant, is essential to some types of meditation, and music is often included in the background of progressive relaxation and visualization tapes.

Music can also help you achieve relaxation on your own, as can natural sounds, for their part. If you can't get to a place where those sounds occur, tapes are available. Even some alarm clocks will enable you to go to sleep and wake up to pleasant sounds. More high-tech sound techniques include hemisync techniques, created by stereo headphones. These sounds are designed to coordinate the left and right hemispheres of the brain.

MEDICATIONS

Medications are standard treatment for many of the conditions that increase stroke risk, including such chronic conditions as hypertension and diabetes mellitus. If you have one of these conditions, taking your prescribed medications can keep your condition under control and significantly reduce that risk. This is something to keep in mind even if you are at low risk for stroke because the incidence of these conditions—and others—increases with age. For people who do not currently have one of these conditions, the role of medication is less significant, although that may change in the future. It depends in part on gender and in part on the outcome of ongoing research. At present, only women stand to benefit from a medication prescribed for something other than a condition that increases stroke risk.

Oral Contraceptives/Hormone Replacement Therapy

As I explain in chapters 3 and 4, estrogen may protect against the type of ischemic stroke caused by atherosclerosis and increase the risk of ischemic stroke caused by embolisms, or clots, that originate in the heart. This female hormone is the primary component of both oral contraceptives and hormone replacement therapy, widely prescribed medications that women take by choice. Your stroke risk profile can help you and your doctor decide whether you should take them or choose another option for birth control or menopausal symptoms and conditions.

If you have any risk factors for atherosclerotic ischemic stroke—say, you have long eaten a high-fat, high-cholesterol diet and have a family history of atherosclerosis—you may afford yourself some additional protection against stroke by choosing oral contraceptives as your form of birth control or hormone replacement therapy to counter your menopausal symptoms. You should know, however, that several recent studies, including preliminary information from the Women's Health Initiative, indicate that estrogen may not have the protective effect observed in other studies. If, however, you have any risk factors for cardioembolic stroke, such as mitral valve disease or atrial fibrillation, you may want to choose another option. Making this choice can prevent the development of an additional risk factor.

Medications That Prevent the Development of Risk Factors

In time, this type of preemptive prevention may extend to more women, including those with the potential for developing other risk factors, as well as to men. As I mention elsewhere, ongoing research has identified what we believe to be a way to predict the development of certain risk factors. We also believe it's possible to prevent some risk factors from developing with medication. I discuss this concept in more detail in chapter 8.

THE PLAN IN PRACTICE

Although you will need your doctor's involvement if you wish to use medications to reduce your risk of stroke, you can incorporate most of the Stroke-Free for Life Plan—and achieve most of its benefits—on your own. This is the most empowering aspect of the plan—and of stroke prevention in general. There is so much that you can do to reduce stroke risk effectively. In fact, some of the most important stroke risk factors are entirely within your control.

If you take my advice and adopt a brain-healthy lifestyle now, while you're at low risk, chances are you will never personally need the information in the rest of the chapters in this book. You'll spare yourself and your loved ones the trauma and disability of stroke, and the arduous work of rehabilitation. Instead, you'll have all the gifts of health that you can possibly bestow on yourself—and many more years to enjoy them!

6

Emergency Treatment for a Brain Attack

Even if you've taken steps to prevent your stroke, there may be risk factors of age, genes, and medical history over which you have little or no control. If you do have a stroke, your understanding of the early warning signs and how to respond to a brain attack in the first critical hours can spell the difference between death and survival, between disability and recovery. In this chapter I'll take you step-by-step through a stroke emergency and highlight your need-to-know stroke survival checklist:

- How to recognize the signs and symptoms of an impending stroke
- Where to go when you have a stroke
- What will happen when you get to the hospital

A TALE OF TWO PATIENTS

Steve was having breakfast with his wife one morning when he felt the left side of his body become weak and numb. He watched helplessly as his coffee cup slipped from his grasp and shattered on the floor. When his wife asked him what was wrong, he moved his mouth to speak, but his tongue wouldn't respond and his speech was unintelligible, even to him. His wife called 911, and moments later was holding his hand in the ambulance on the way to the emergency room.

Steve was diagnosed with acute ischemic stroke and, within ninety minutes of his arrival, treated with thrombolytic (clot-busting) therapy. By the next day, his numbness had turned to a faint weakness, and his speech was returning to normal. Two months later, he had no lasting effects of his stroke and was on a diet, exercise, and medication regimen to prevent a recurrence.

When Martha experienced similar symptoms one morning, she didn't call the doctor. She had experienced brief periods of weakness on her left side during the previous weeks, and they had faded away within minutes. She figured her latest episode would disappear on its own if she just lay down and rested. Maybe it was just bad circulation. Part of getting older.

As the hours went by, her symptoms worsened. She couldn't lift her left arm at all. When her husband came home from work that evening, he was alarmed to discover that she couldn't sit up straight on the sofa. He insisted that she go to the hospital. Ten hours had passed since the onset of her first symptoms.

Martha was diagnosed with ischemic stroke. Since she had waited all day to seek help, it wasn't possible to give her the thrombolytic treatment that Steve had received. Instead, she was given medication to stop the damage from progressing and to prevent a recurrence. After weeks of physical therapy, she was able to walk again—with the aid of a cane—but she has never regained the use of her left arm.

Steve and his wife realized that stroke is a medical emergency and responded accordingly. Martha did not. Her lack of information about what was happening to her brain and body cost her dearly. A formerly active woman in her mid-sixties, she and her husband are now facing a life of diminished function and compromised fulfillment. Instead of low-impact aerobics, she's in rehab. She used to ice-skate with her seven-year-old granddaughter on Wednesday afternoons and go birding with her husband most weekends. Now she's relearning how to write a grocery list.

Martha's inaction in the face of a brain attack is tragically commonplace. According to a recent Gallup Survey conducted for the National Stroke Association, only 40 percent of adults age fifty or older said they would call 911 immediately if they were having a stroke. Though most elderly people live in dread of a stroke, few of them know that stroke can be treated. It's true that, until recently, there was little we could do for a person who was having a stroke. But that's no longer the case. In the last decade or so, major lifesaving advances have transformed the treatment of ischemic stroke. The most exciting of these advances, thrombolytic therapy, has the potential significantly to reduce major disability and save the lives of victims of ischemic stroke.

Thrombolytic therapy is a highly time-sensitive treatment. When given intravenously, it is effective only when administered within the first three hours after ischemic stroke symptoms appear. After that, it may do more harm than good. In fact, its effectiveness dwindles even within the three-hour window, which makes every minute count. People who don't seek immediate medical attention—or who go to an ill-equipped hospital—will miss out on one of the most profound medical advances in a generation.

Stroke is a medical emergency. How you respond in those first few moments—or at most, the first few hours—could make a crucial difference to your longevity, and to the quality of your life for years, or even decades, to come. There are dramatic new treatments at your fingertips, but unless you know when, how, and where to reach out and grasp them, you are likely to fumble away your best chance of continued health. You and I could try to fault others for insufficient efforts to educate the public about stroke emergencies and make state-of-the-art acute stroke treatment available at every hospital day and night. That wouldn't change the fact that for now, the key to saving *your* life's productivity or that of a loved one depends on *your* preparation for a stroke crisis, and *your* ability to take swift and decisive action.

RECOGNIZING THE SIGNS AND SYMPTOMS

First, you need to recognize the signs and symptoms of stroke. This is important for prevention as well as for treatment. Some signs indicate not that stroke has occurred but that it is highly likely (Martha's earlier, temporary periods of weakness, for instance). Recognizing and acting on these signs could prevent a stroke. Other signs indicate that a stroke is occurring and that you need to seek medical attention immediately.

Stroke symptoms vary depending on the cause, location, and severity of the brain injury. Reporting the symptoms you've experienced or are experiencing to your doctor can give him or her a head start in diagnosis and treatment. Recognizing stroke signs and symptoms early is your best shot at early treatment—and early treatment of stroke can mean the difference between life and death, between severe disability and minor disability or no disability at all.

What follows is a list of possible stroke symptoms. If you're experiencing a stroke, chances are you will not experience all of the symptoms. If you experience any of these symptoms, especially in combination, you should seek medical attention immediately.

- **Sudden numbness, weakness, or paralysis of the face, arm, or leg,** usually on only one side of the body.
- **Sudden difficulty speaking or trouble understanding others.** This includes the inability to articulate correctly (dysarthria), impaired ability to produce sound (dysphonia), and the loss of the ability to produce or comprehend spoken or written language (dysphasia).
- **Sudden blurred or decreased vision, loss of vision, or double vision.** This includes the sudden loss of vision in one eye or both eyes, visual impairment in only one eye, and visual impairment of the left or right field of vision in one or both eyes.
- **Sudden dizziness, loss of balance, or loss of coordination.**
- **Sudden, severe headache.** This pain, which is sometimes described as "like being hit over the head with a hammer," may be accompanied by a stiff neck, facial pain, pain between the eyes, vomiting, or altered consciousness. This combination indicates the possibility of hemorrhagic stroke.
- **Sudden cognitive abnormalities.** These can include problems with memory, spatial orientation, and perception.
- **Seizures or loss of consciousness.** Seizures, spells of abnormal neurological function, can be associated with stroke, as can transient loss of consciousness, for example, fainting or blacking out. Neither of these signs is commonly linked to stroke, though.

Keeping these signs and symptoms in mind, particularly if you or a loved one is at risk of stroke, will enable you to take prompt action when they occur—action that could save your life and productivity.

WHERE TO GO FOR HELP

Your choice of a hospital for acute stroke treatment is almost as important to your overall health outcome as is your ability to recognize the signs and symptoms of stroke. Although emergency stroke treatment has improved tremendously in the last decade, not all hospitals are equipped to treat acute stroke.

Most hospitals have computed tomography (CT) or magnetic resonance imaging (MRI) scanners, but this equipment may not be available twenty-four hours a day on an emergency basis. Or the hospital may not always have a radiologist available to interpret the results. These imaging tests are needed for the rapid diagnosis of stroke, including stroke type. Since the clot-busting thrombolytic therapy that could save the productive life of a person suffering an ischemic stroke could *increase* bleeding in a person suffering a hemorrhagic stroke—with potentially fatal results—diagnosis of stroke type is crucial for treatment.

Even if a hospital has the ability to determine quickly that you are suffering an acute ischemic stroke, it may not be able to offer state-of-the-art treatment. Thrombolytic therapy is fairly new. Only an estimated 25 to 35 percent of the nation's hospitals have the ability to deliver it. The percentage may be even lower in your area. What's more, a recent study indicates that some of the hospitals that offer the therapy aren't giving it to many of the patients who are eligible or are giving it after the three-hour window has passed. If you go to a hospital that doesn't offer thrombolytic therapy, the three-hour time window may very well pass before you can get to another hospital.

Another important consideration is location. Even the best-equipped hospital is of little help if it's three hundred miles away. Intravenous thrombolytic therapy has to be administered within three hours after the onset of stroke symptoms. If you have to travel hours to get to the hospital, you'll miss that critical treatment window.

I believe that the number of hospitals that can deliver state-of-the-art treatment will steadily increase over time—but since location and access to imaging tests and thrombolytic therapy can limit your choices, you need to plan ahead. Research the hospitals in your area and decide, *in advance of an emergency,* which hospital you should go to if you experience stroke symptoms. In chapter 9, "A Stroke Survival Manual," I provide you with more detailed criteria to evaluate the hospitals in your area. You should perform this evaluation sooner rather than later. If you wait until you have a stroke, it will be too late. I don't want to alarm you, but I do want you to be prepared. So please, read chapter 9 as soon as you've completed this chapter.

Once you've identified the hospital you would go to in a stroke emergency, write the name and address down and keep the information in your wallet. That way, when you call 911, you can tell the operator or the ambulance personnel where to take you. In the rush of a medical emergency, when you may not have all your faculties at your command, you'll need to have this important information close at hand.

THE FIRST STEPS IN ACUTE STROKE TREATMENT

Let's assume you've done your homework. You've identified a qualified medical center near you, you're familiar with the various stroke symptoms, and you've called 911 immediately after you've experienced them. What should you expect when you get to the hospital you've chosen? In the rest of this chapter, I walk you through the ins and outs of acute stroke treatment.

The better informed you are about what to expect during emergency stroke treatment, the more helpful you'll be to the hospital staff that's working to save your brain. Also, if you know what to expect, you'll be more relaxed and cooperative, which is no small feat during any medical emergency. The success of emergency stroke treatment hinges on a doctor's ability to assess quickly the type and location of your stroke. A correct diagnosis depends on having good technology available, a well-trained doctor examining you, and your ability to follow directions and offer helpful information during the exam.

Diagnosis

The first step in treating stroke, as with virtually any condition, is accurate diagnosis. To treat stroke, your doctor needs to know with as much certainty as possible that a stroke has occurred and what type of stroke it is. He or she also must establish the time that its symptoms began. This diagnosis is crucial. You cannot be sure you're beginning optimum treatment without it. Diagnosis involves a number of steps—more in some cases than in others—but certain steps are performed first in most cases to avoid delay and ensure that treatment can begin as soon as possible.

When you arrive at the hospital, you can expect your doctor to:

1. take a directed medical history to find out about your symptoms and when and how they began;
2. perform a directed physical examination that includes a neurological component;
3. order an urgent computed tomography, or CT, scan to determine if you're having an ischemic or hemorrhagic stroke; and
4. order a series of laboratory tests, including blood tests to measure the levels of blood glucose, electrolytes, and oxygen in the blood, a blood test for the presence of creatinine, which indicates kidney function, and a complete blood count.

Your doctor may also order a chest X ray and electrocardiogram (EKG).

Although this may sound like a lengthy process, it's not. These diagnostic components are performed rapidly, either one right after the other or simultaneously. The goal is to determine as quickly as possible whether you are having a stroke, what kind of stroke you are having, and whether you would benefit from emergency treatment like thrombolytic therapy. Additional tests may follow before or after treatment is administered if diagnostic questions remain.

Let's step back now and take a closer look at these and other tests and procedures so you can get a better idea of what to expect.

History

When you arrive at the hospital, the doctor will ask questions about the symptoms that brought you to the hospital, including when they started, how quickly they started, and whether they've gotten better, worse, or stayed the same. Answer these questions accurately and with as much detail as possible. Your answers will help the doctor determine if you are having a stroke, what type of stroke you are having, and what type of treatment you should receive. The doctor will also take your medical history, looking for any risk factors you may have. For example, he or she may ask about the condition of your heart, whether you have hypertension, whether you've had a transient ischemic attack, and whether you smoke.

EXAMINATION

By this time, the examination will already be under way. Since the exam begins with general neurological observations, the doctor will have noted certain things while he or she was taking your history. If you had difficulty remembering what happened to you or putting your experience into words, for example, the doctor will have taken note. He or she may also have observed your body, including the way your arms and legs are positioned, the way you move, and the appearance of your skin. These factors can give clues about whether you've had a stroke, what part of the brain is affected, and what the underlying mechanism might be.

The observational portion of the exam—as well as the physical portion that follows—varies from person to person, depending on the symptoms displayed and the order in which the doctor chooses to conduct the examination. An experienced physician can conduct this exam quite rapidly. Here is an idea of some of the things that you might expect to happen. The doctor may:

- Test the muscle strength in your arms, legs, and face and watch as you turn your head, raise your arm, and walk, noticing any muscle weakness as well as your posture and gait.
- Check to see if you can feel various sensory stimuli in different parts of your body.
- Examine your eyes and ask you to participate in some visual tests. Although you might think these exercises seem unrelated to stroke, the eyes can often help the doctor "see" what's going on in the brain. Certain eye movements, pupil reactions, and visual deficits suggest problems in certain parts of the brain, and abnormalities of the blood vessels of the eye can indicate vascular problems elsewhere in the body.
- Observe the inside of your mouth as you open and say, "Ah," to see if the parts of the brain that govern speaking and swallowing have been affected.
- Check for difficulties of language function and difficulties of speech. You may be asked to repeat a word or sentence, to name various objects, or to write various letters, numbers, or words, for example.

- Test your deep tendon reflexes.
- Place a stethoscope over your heart, then move up the shoulders and neck into the head to listen for sounds, or "bruits," from the arteries that carry blood to the brain.
- Check the pulse in various arteries in the head to estimate blood flow through the arteries that supply the brain.

In order to find out as much as possible about the current condition of your body, the doctor will also listen to your heart, take your pulse and blood pressure, listen to your breathing, and examine your head, chest, and abdomen. All of these tests can help the doctor determine the location of the stroke and the extent of the damage.

Despite all the things your doctor is checking, the examination takes place relatively quickly. Indeed, for ischemic stroke treatment to occur within three hours, it has to. During this time, the doctor will order several blood tests and an imaging test—computed tomography or magnetic resonance imaging—which may actually precede the examination.

TESTS

To ensure an accurate diagnosis of stroke type, the doctor needs a picture of your brain tissue.

CT scan

The imaging test most commonly used for this purpose is the CT scan, which uses multiple rotating beams of X rays to create a cross-sectional picture of the brain. A CT scan can confirm the presence of most hemorrhages, define the location and size of the injured area, and help identify the location and size of an area injured by ischemic stroke. Damage caused by ischemic stroke usually does not show up on a CT scan right away. If the area of damage is small or located in the back part of the brain, it may not show up at all. As a result, CT is most effective for quickly diagnosing—or ruling out—hemorrhagic stroke. It can enable the doctor to see the bleeding and, in many cases, to find the source of the bleeding, a ruptured aneurysm or vascular malformation, for example.

MRI

Another imaging test you may encounter, on its own or in conjunction with CT, is MRI, which uses magnetic fields and radio-frequency pulses to create images. The images MRI produces are usually more detailed than those produced by CT. MRI images may pick up small areas of damage, particularly in certain areas of the brain, that CT may miss. The drawback to MRI is that you have to lie still inside an enclosed scanner for approximately thirty minutes. That's longer than a CT scan takes, and the tight enclosure of the MRI scanner can cause claustrophobia for some people.

Blood Tests

Other tests you will undergo early on are blood tests. These will likely include measures of blood glucose (a type of sugar), electrolytes (substances in the blood such as sodium and potassium), creatinine (a metabolic substance used to measure kidney function), and a complete blood count, or CBC, which measures levels of hemoglobin (a protein-iron compound in the blood that carries oxygen), platelets (small components of blood essential for clotting), and hematocrit (an index of the number of cells in the blood). The hematocrit count helps indicate how easily blood flows. Another test that indicates this is blood viscosity, which measures the thickness of the blood. Fibrinogen, another component of blood that aids in clotting, may also be measured. The blood itself may be tested to see how long it takes to clot, through tests such as partial thromboplastin time, bleeding time, and prothrombin time. Pulse oximetry may be used to measure the level of oxygen saturation in the blood.

Electrocardiography and echocardiography

Your doctor may also order electrocardiography (you may know this test as an ECG or EKG) and a chest X-ray to produce an image of the heart. If a cardiac problem is suspected as the source of an ischemic stroke, additional tests, like echocardiography (a form of ultrasound used to produce an image of the heart and assess its function), may be ordered. This may play a crucial role in determining the type of emergency treatment you receive, because ischemic stroke treatment with thrombolytic therapy rules out immediate treatment with anticoagulants, and vice versa.

Coupled with the history and exam, these tests and an imaging test often provide enough information to make a diagnosis and begin treatment. In some situations, other tests may be needed. The value of these tests must be weighed against the cost of delaying treatment, particularly when it comes to thrombolytic treatment of ischemic stroke. In other cases, the tests may be administered after thrombolytic therapy is delivered.

Other tests

Some of the additional tests you may undergo depending on your situation include imaging tests designed to assess the blood vessels and blood flow. These tests include various types of **ultrasound,** which uses sound waves to create images, and **magnetic resonance angiography, or MRA,** a variation of MRI used to image the vascular system. To obtain an ultrasound image, the doctor or a technician places a cigar-shaped instrument called a transducer over the arteries in question to record sounds. Variations include **Doppler testing,** which measures how fast blood flows through the vessels; **B-mode imaging,** which shows the type and severity of structural arterial changes; and **duplex scanning,** which combines B-mode imaging and Doppler testing. MRA may be performed when either hemorrhagic or ischemic stroke is suspected. It helps the doctor visualize the blood vessels in the head to determine the cause of the hemorrhage or infarct and what type of treatment is most appropriate.

A lower-tech test that can offer important information about your circulation is **ocular pneumoplethysgraphy, or OPG.** This test measures the blood pressure in the eye. It can effectively show a major blockage in either carotid system. Unlike ultrasound, it covers the entire carotid system. It is also less expensive.

Another test that can pinpoint problems in the arteries is **arteriography.** In this more invasive test, a dye is injected into a suspect artery and then X rays are taken. This process makes the arteries—and such problems as a bleeding aneurysm or an arteriovenous malformation—visible. It is required if the doctor intends to deliver thrombolytic therapy directly to an artery, a procedure that is being used in some medical centers. Arteriography is also required if an endovascular procedure like coiling (threading a catheter to the area to deliver a coil into the aneurysm to prevent its rupture) is going to be used as a treatment for subarachnoid or intracerebral hemorrhage. In fact, in these cases, it is the first step of the procedure. Arteriography is the gold standard for determining what is going on in the blood vessels, but it carries a slight risk of stroke, so it's not performed unless it can provide vital information.

Other tests that are occasionally ordered either immediately or soon after stroke include **electroencephalography,** which measures the electrical activity in the brain and can occasionally help locate the damage caused by stroke or any associated seizure activity. On rare occasions, if CT and MRI are inconclusive or unavailable, or if the doctor suspects subarachnoid hemorrhage or meningitis, he or she may order a **lumbar puncture, or spinal tap.** This test, which involves inserting a needle into the lower spine to obtain a small amount of cerebrospinal fluid from the spine for study, can usually identify whether a stroke is hemorrhagic or ischemic.

Emergency Treatment

As you might expect, the techniques I've just described have made it much easier to diagnose stroke quickly and accurately, but though the diagnosis is quick, it isn't instantaneous. While you're undergoing examinations and tests, something is going wrong in your brain, and possibly in your heart and other areas of your body. Although we can't administer certain treatments until we have the results of diagnostic tests, we don't simply ignore your physical condition while we wait. We do what we can to make sure that you're breathing adequately, that your heart is functioning adequately, and that you remain as stable as possible until we know more definitively what type of stroke you're experiencing and can take action to treat it.

Regardless of the type of stroke, your doctor's first priority is to make sure you are getting enough air. This is particularly important if you have a respiratory problem or if you are unconscious. The doctor may suction your airway, administer supplemental oxygen, and place you in a lateral position to facilitate breathing if necessary. The doctor will also pay special attention to your cardiovascular system, treating any general circulatory problems he or she finds. This could include treating shock, controlling rhythm disorders, and administering medication to treat heart failure. Careful monitoring of body temperature and treatment of fever are also important. Your doctor may also need to reduce your blood pressure, particularly if you are suffering from a heart attack, heart failure, acute kidney failure, or your pressure is high and you are receiving thrombolytic therapy, but he or she must do it gradually. Lowering blood pressure too quickly can result in even less blood flow to areas of the brain where blood is already in short supply.

The doctor will also monitor your intake of fluids and your electrolytes to make sure they remain in balance. If you show signs of swelling that places pressure on the brain, the doctor may order one of several treatments to reduce that pressure, which could otherwise be fatal. These treatments could include such simple procedures as raising the head of the bed and restricting fluid intake; such medications as diuretics, mannitol, glycerol, and steroids; and, rarely, such interventional procedures as hemicraniectomy (removal of part of half of the skull), decompression, and ventricular drainage (creating an opening to allow fluid and blood to drain from the ventricles of the brain).

TREATING ACUTE ISCHEMIC STROKE

Let's assume that your test results indicate that you've had an ischemic stroke. Several treatment options are available to you. Your doctor will choose one based on your condition, the severity of the stroke you've experienced, and when your symptoms began.

Thrombolytic Therapy: The Clot Busters

If your doctor has diagnosed you with an ischemic stroke and you've reported to the hospital within three hours of when your symptoms began, you may be a candidate for intravenous thrombolytic therapy. Also known as clot-busting therapy, thrombolytic therapy involves injecting a drug into a vein (or artery) to dissolve blood clots and to restore blood flow to the brain. Thrombolytic therapy can significantly reduce neurological damage and save lives—but only if it is administered correctly and in a timely fashion.

Thrombolytic medications, tissue plasminogen activator (tPA), for example, can cause bleeding in the brain or cause a hemorrhage to worsen, sometimes with fatal results. As a result, they should not be given to anyone who is experiencing a hemorrhagic stroke or who has risk factors for hemorrhage. If thrombolytic medications are given intravenously, as they most often are, they should be given within three hours of the onset of stroke symptoms, and they should be given only to people who are experiencing a moderate or severe ischemic stroke with symptoms that are not rapidly improving.

Recent studies indicate that the effectiveness of thrombolytic therapy is directly related to when it is administered. The sooner it is given, the better the patient's recovery. Thrombolytic drugs are generally not used for people in a coma, people experiencing seizures, people with a history of intracranial hemorrhage, people whose blood pressure is consistently more than 185/110 mm Hg, and people who have had a recent internal hemorrhage, for example, a hemorrhage in the gastrointestinal or urinary tracts. Likewise, they are generally not used for people who have had another major ischemic stroke within the past two weeks, people who have been treated with the anticoagulant heparin within forty-eight hours, and people whose blood is too thin and slow to clot.

Just how important those criteria are was recently underscored by the results of a study of stroke patients in twenty-nine hospitals in a major metropolitan area treated with tPA. Researchers found that doctors did not follow the recommended guidelines for administering tPA in about 50 percent of cases. Possibly as a result, 15.7 percent of the patients treated with tPA experienced bleeding in the brain, and more than half of these individuals died from the bleeding. The overall death rate for patients given tPA was 15.7 percent, compared with 5.1 percent in stroke patients who did not receive the treatment.

If tPA is administered according to guidelines, the results are much more favorable. Four major studies have found that between 31 and 50 percent of patients given the treatment within three hours of the onset of ischemic stroke symptoms had a complete or near-complete recovery, compared with 20 to 38 percent of patients given a placebo, or inactive, treatment. Brain hemorrhage occurred in between 6.4 and 8 percent of treated patients, as opposed to 0.6 to 2.4 percent of those given a placebo.

These studies underscore just how important it is to choose a hospital with experienced and well-trained stroke emergency staff. It doesn't matter how good the technology may be at any given hospital if the medical personnel don't understand how and when to administer thrombolytic therapy.

Anticoagulant and Antiplatelet Medications:
The Blood Thinners

If you are not a candidate for tPA, other medications are available to treat acute ischemic stroke. Anticoagulants and antiplatelet agents—drugs used to prevent ischemic stroke in certain at-risk people—are also used to treat ischemic stroke when it occurs. As I explained in chapter 3, these medications, sometimes called blood thinners, work by reducing the blood's tendency to coagulate. They prevent the formation of additional clots, prevent existing clots from growing, and enable blood to flow more freely through narrowed arteries.

The choice of blood-thinning drugs depends on a number of factors, including the cause, location, and severity of the ischemic stroke and the patient's general health. The most powerful and fast-acting of these drugs, heparin, is sometimes given to people experiencing ischemic strokes who are not candidates for thrombolytic therapy. If you arrived at the hospital more than three hours after your symptoms began, for example, your doctor may recommend treatment with heparin. This anticoagulant, which is given intravenously, takes effect almost immediately. It is particularly useful in treating people whose ischemic strokes are cardiac in origin and those in whom a condition that makes clotting more likely (for instance, a blood disorder like antiphospholipid antibody syndrome) is suspected. It is often used to treat patients with mild ischemic stroke and transient ischemic attack.

Because heparin improves the flow of blood and helps prevent clotting, it has the potential to trigger hemorrhage, particularly in people who have developed large infarcts (areas of dead tissue), which may occur, for instance, as a result of a clot that originated in the heart. Heparin generally should not be given to anyone with a bleeding peptic ulcer, liver failure, extremely high blood pressure, or other conditions that may predispose a person to hemorrhage.

Since heparin and other related drugs known as heparinoids are the fastest-acting of the blood-thinning drugs, they are the ones used most often to treat acute ischemic stroke. Slower-acting anticoagulants, like warfarin or dicumarol, may be used to treat minor stroke or TIA but are often given after heparin. These drugs, too, carry risks of hemorrhage. For people who cannot take anticoagulants, such antiplatelet drugs as aspirin, clopidogrel

(Plavix), or Aggrenox (a combination of aspirin and dipyridamole) may be the preferred initial treatment for ischemic stroke or TIA. These medications also play a major role in the continuing treatment of ischemic stroke regardless of severity. I discuss them in more detail in the next chapter.

Neuroprotective Agents: Armor for the Brain

One other type of medication may be at your doctor's disposal to treat acute ischemic stroke—the neuroprotective agents. As their name implies, these medications may protect areas of the brain from permanent damage if they're given shortly after stroke symptoms begin. Exactly how they do this depends on the type of drug used. Some of these medications have been used successfully to treat subarachnoid hemorrhage. Although studies to date have not found that these drugs benefit people with acute ischemic stroke, ongoing studies at stroke treatment centers are examining the effectiveness of several types of neuroprotective medications for treating acute ischemic stroke, particularly in conjunction with thrombolytic agents.

The most familiar of these medications are the calcium channel blockers. This class of drugs, which includes nimodipine, is usually used to treat hypertension. The drugs' ability to block the influx of calcium into cells plays a different role in ischemic stroke. During stroke, excess calcium floods brain cells, causing them to die. By blocking this influx of calcium, calcium channel blockers may save the brain cells from death. Another class of drugs that may block the influx of calcium into brain cells are the N-methyl-D-aspartate (NMDA) antagonists, which include the drugs dextromethorphan and dizocilpine. Free radical scavengers are another class of neuroprotective agents. These drugs are believed to decrease damage to brain cells by "mopping up" free radicals, potentially dangerous unstable oxygen compounds created by the reaction of oxygen and other molecules. Although none of these neuroprotective drugs is in widespread use for the treatment of acute ischemic stroke, you may encounter them if you seek treatment at a medical center that is involved in clinical studies of the drugs.

Emergency Intervention: High-Tech Options

Another treatment option for acute ischemic stroke is emergency intervention. Carotid endarterectomy and carotid angioplasty, preventive treatments I described in chapter 3, are occasionally used as emergency treatments for ischemic stroke, though neither of these procedures has been widely studied for use in this capacity.

Other high-tech interventions include such endovascular procedures as intra-arterial tPA. This variation of conventional thrombolytic therapy is being studied in some specialized medical centers. It involves threading a catheter from the femoral artery into the head to the artery in which a clot has lodged and delivering tPA directly to the clot. In some cases, this is performed in addition to intravenous thrombolytic therapy. Needless to say, this is a complex procedure that can be performed only by a highly skilled individual. It may expand the treatment window for thrombolytic treatment.

Although expanding the treatment window could clearly help save lives, we have not yet fully realized the potential of existing treatments. Currently, only 2 to 3 percent of people with ischemic stroke—approximately 15,000—receive thrombolytic therapy each year. This is partly because most people don't realize that they need to get to the hospital quickly when they experience stroke symptoms. Research indicates that only 15 percent of people suffering from ischemic strokes arrive at the hospital within three hours. In addition, not all hospitals are equipped to deliver thrombolytic therapy. As a result, far fewer people are receiving the drug than can benefit from it.

As more people learn about stroke and more hospitals add the technology, this will change. Theoretically, about half of all people with ischemic strokes—300,000 each year—could potentially undergo the therapy, although logistics will undoubtedly keep us from treating all possible patients. Of those, approximately 15 percent will receive major life-altering benefits from the therapy, which translates into tens of thousands more patients each year.

TREATING ACUTE HEMORRHAGIC STROKE

If you've been diagnosed with hemorrhagic stroke, your initial treatment will differ from what I just described. The treatment you receive will depend on the type of hemorrhagic stroke you are experiencing, the severity of the stroke, and other factors.

Subarachnoid Hemorrhage

If you've experienced a subarachnoid hemorrhage, your early treatment will largely be aimed at preventing and managing such neurological complications as rebleeding of an aneurysm, vasospasm (a spasm that narrows blood vessels), ischemic stroke, hydrocephalus (an accumulation of fluid and pressure in the brain), and seizures (episodes of sudden, involuntary muscle contractions).

To prevent an aneurysm from bleeding again, your doctor may place you on bed rest in a quiet room, elevate the head of your bed, and keep you under close observation. You may be given stool softeners and cough suppressants to keep you from straining, pain relievers to control any pain, and a mild sedative if you are agitated and cannot remain quiet and still. If your blood pressure is extremely high, you may be given medications to reduce it.

Perhaps the most important action your doctor can take to prevent rebleeding is to clip or coil the aneurysm or correct the vascular (blood vessel) malformation that has ruptured. I describe these procedures in detail in chapter 4. Briefly, clipping involves isolating the aneurysm from the blood supply by placing a clip across its neck. If that is not feasible, a catheter can be threaded through to the area to deliver a coil into the aneurysm to prevent its rupture. These surgical procedures should take place as soon as possible if the person is in good condition. They generally take place within the first three days after the stroke occurs, but the actual timing may vary. Surgery may be immediate if rebleeding has already occurred. Vascular malformations can be removed surgically or corrected with any of a number of endovascular procedures.

Your doctor will also take steps to prevent vasospasm, a natural defense mechanism in which the arteries, in the face of blood outside the artery, go into spasm and narrow, which restricts the flow of blood and oxygen to the brain and sometimes results in ischemic stroke. For starters, your doctor will make sure that you are getting the right amount of fluids and electrolytes, because dehydration can lead to vasospasm. You may also be given a calcium channel blocking drug like nimodipine, which can help prevent smooth muscles, like those in the arteries, from contracting. If you are among the 30 percent of people with subarachnoid hemorrhage who do experience vasospasm, your doctor may administer a medication or blood product to expand the volume of your blood.

Another potential complication of subarachnoid hemorrhage is hydrocephalus. Commonly known as water on the brain, hydrocephalus is actually an accumulation of cerebrospinal fluid in the ventricles of the brain, which places pressure on the brain. This condition, which affects approximately 20 percent of people with subarachnoid hemorrhage, may resolve on its own. If it causes neurological impairments, your doctor may treat it with a surgical procedure in which he or she places a drain in the brain to allow the fluid to exit the body.

One further neurological complication of subarachnoid hemorrhage is seizures, which occur in approximately 3 to 5 percent of patients. If you are one of them, your doctor may treat you with a short-acting seizure control drug such as diazepam followed by a longer-acting antiseizure medication.

Intracerebral Hemorrhage

If you've suffered an intracerebral hemorrhage, your doctor will evaluate you to determine whether you should receive emergency surgery. Generally, surgery is recommended for people who have experienced a moderate to large hemorrhage and show mild signs that their brain stem is being compressed or affected. Depending on the location and size of the hemorrhage, emergency surgery could include draining the hematoma, or pool of blood, that has accumulated in the brain and is increasing pressure on the brain. It could also include clipping or coiling a ruptured aneurysm or removing a blood vessel malformation to stop the bleeding and prevent it from recurring.

If you are not a surgical candidate, your doctor will treat you medically. The three-part treatment strategy includes relieving pressure and swelling of the brain with drugs such as mannitol or glycerol, steroids, or sometimes urgent intubation and induced rapid breathing; controlling blood pressure; and maintaining the proper balance of fluids and electrolytes. In addition, the doctor will likely place you on bed rest, elevate the head of your bed, restrict fluids, and have you closely monitored. You may be given stool softeners and cough medication to prevent straining, medication to relieve pain, and a mild sedative if you are agitated. You also may be treated with anticonvulsants if you experience seizures. Sometimes intracerebral hemorrhage and subarachnoid hemorrhage coexist. In these cases, other treatments, like those described above for vasospasm, may be useful.

THE TAKE-AWAY LESSON FROM THIS CHAPTER

As you can see, state-of-the-art emergency stroke treatment involves high technology, a vast array of treatment options, and highly trained medical personnel. Since you can't expect to be as expert as the doctors in this crisis, your most important role is as an informed health consumer—choosing the right hospital to go to. After that, you have to put yourself into the hands of the experts you've chosen.

Even under the best of circumstances—the best medical center and the best doctors—you can never predict the outcome from a brain attack. Which is why prevention remains your best option.

WHAT COMES NEXT

Although treatment of acute stroke plays a crucial role in whether you will live or die and whether you will have any lasting deficits, ongoing treatment is equally important to your health. It can help prevent stroke from recurring with more serious consequences, and it can help you recover from or regain any abilities you lost as a result of the stroke. The next chapter deals with the ongoing treatment of stroke.

7

Assessing and Treating Damage from a Brain Attack

In many ways, one can think of a brain attack like a military episode similar to a submarine attack on a battleship. First, there is the unexpected impact of an unseen missile that blows a hole in the ship's hull. Initial panic is replaced by emergency response as the crew moves quickly to regain control of the ship. Hatches are sealed, water bailed. The captain receives damage reports from all decks and decides how to defend the ship and fend off further attacks. Then the captain directs the ship to the nearest safe harbor to begin repairs.

In the previous chapter, I've detailed what happens in the hospital during the critical hours following a brain attack. This emergency treatment is literally first aid: the first—not the final—stage of treatment. Acute stroke treatment, like other medical first aid, may save your life and reduce the amount of damage to your brain. The treatment that follows is what will address the damage that has occurred, protect you from another attack, and help restore and rehabilitate you to the greatest extent possible.

I've drawn this battleship analogy because repairing and rehabilitating the damage from a brain attack involves the efforts of many medical personnel from many disciplines, not to mention family and friends. I hasten to add that a stroke victim is not a battleship or a car or any other machine. Human beings are much more complex than any man-made object, and the human brain is the most intricate of all organisms. Recovering from a stroke involves rehabilitating the body, the mind, the emotions, the senses—even the soul. Although a stroke is technically an assault on the brain, its damage can manifest in every aspect of consciousness.

The good news is that as humans, we can draw on all of our strengths—physical, psychological, and spiritual—to aid in our recovery. Let me give you just one, extraordinary example.

Billy was a high school football star who everyone predicted was headed for athletic glory as a wide receiver at the college and, perhaps, professional level. During the final game of his junior year, he caught a pass in the end zone, was upended by an opponent, and landed on his head. Dazed by the fall, he managed to stagger off the field to the applause of his teammates and fans.

What Billy didn't know was that the trauma to his neck caused a dissection of his carotid artery. The inner lining of the arterial wall in his neck folded in on itself and a clot formed there. Two hours after the end of the game, the clot traveled upstream to his brain, causing an ischemic stroke. By the next morning, he was referred to Mayo. When I examined him in the hospital, he had trouble speaking and moving the right side of his body. The MRI revealed the culprit: a left cerebral infarct.

The days that followed were intensely sad and emotionally trying for his family, his friends and classmates, and of course, most of all, for Billy. When he realized that he could have lasting deficits, he was understandably quite depressed and anxious. He could easily have lost hope and given in to despair. I watched in amazement as this young man picked himself up and marched bravely into rehabilitation. I don't know what well of internal strength he drew from—his experience in athletic training, his spiritual focus, or simply his strength of character—but over the ensuing months he gave us all a lesson in courage.

The only direct medical aid was the blood-thinning drugs we put him on to prevent further clots from forming. Fortunately, his condition, called a carotid dissection, was able to heal itself over time. The rehabilitation he achieved was hard work. Speech therapy overcame his language difficulties after a couple of months, and various physical therapies enabled him to recover normal function after six to eight months.

The summer before his senior year, Billy told me he wanted to resume competitive sports. Football was out of the question, but he was a natural athlete, and he was able to make the transition to track and field. After training all fall, he not only made the team, but he became a co-captain. That spring, he competed in the statewide championships and won a medal in the high jump.

Billy's is a truly heroic story, but it has relevance to anyone facing rehabilitation from stroke. You may be dependent on a lot of people for help, and you may not recover all the functions lost to stroke. But no one can set limits for you. It's up to you to decide on your goals and move toward them. A stroke may rob you of the full use of your body or mind—but it can't take away your spirit or your will to recover. Time and again, I've watched patients overcome enormous obstacles, both medical and psychological, to regain their dignity and control over their lives.

THE STAGES OF STROKE TREATMENT AND REHABILITATION

The distinction between acute stroke treatment and the treatment that follows is one of time and context. Although we generally consider acute stroke treatment to be treatment that occurs within the first twenty-four hours of the appearance of stroke symptoms, we can and often do progress from a treatment that is considered acute to one that is considered subacute before twenty-four hours have passed. Likewise, if a person doesn't report to the hospital until days after he or she began experiencing stroke symptoms, that person would undergo some procedures—including diagnosis—that are normally performed in the acute phase well after that twenty-four-hour phase is over. In other words, there's no magical point at which care moves beyond the acute stage.

With that in mind, this chapter focuses on the treatment and care that is given when the actual brain attack is complete—usually twenty-four hours or more after symptoms began—and the context has switched from preventing damage to assessing and addressing the damage that has occurred. Specifically, I'll be taking you through the following medical treatment stages:

1. Assessing damage
2. Preventing and addressing complications

3. Treating underlying causes and preventing recurrent stroke
4. Rehabilitation

ASSESSING DAMAGE

Your doctor begins assessing the damage caused by your stroke when you first come into the emergency room for diagnosis. The physical examination he or she performs, particularly the neurological component, provides a good idea of the extent of damage the brain has sustained and where that damage is located. Likewise, the imaging tests the doctor performs during diagnosis indicate the location, type, and extent of the damage. I discuss these diagnostic procedures in detail in chapter 6.

Assessment does not end with diagnosis. For one thing, not all damage shows up immediately on imaging tests. Depending on when the scan is taken, computed tomography, or CT, produces negative results in up to 50 percent of ischemic strokes within the first twenty-four hours. It is more likely to be negative immediately after the stroke. For another, some deficits that initially may be present may resolve with time. For these reasons, and the fact that your overall condition may change on its own or as a result of treatment, your doctor may continue to perform and, in many cases, repeat assessment tests for several weeks. Here's a taste of what you can expect.

Physical/Neurologic Examinations

You should expect to be examined regularly. As a stroke survivor, you've just come through a serious health emergency, and your doctor needs to monitor your overall health, watch for the development of complications, and assess the damage caused by your stroke. As I've said, the deficits caused by stroke sometimes take time to appear and sometimes resolve on their own. Repeated neurological exams can help the doctor determine what deficits you currently have. I explain the examination procedure in chapter 6. To refresh your memory, it may include observation of, questions about, and assessments of your movement, reflexes and coordination, speech and communication skills, sensory abilities, ophthalmologic exams, and examinations of the cranial nerves. It also includes such standard examination procedures as monitoring your heart and blood pressure.

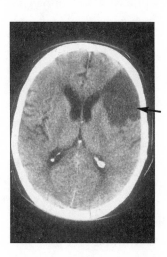

A computed tomography (CT) scan of the head (horizontal cut) shows a moderately large left cerebral infarct, or ischemic stroke (dark area shown by arrow), in the frontal region three days after onset.

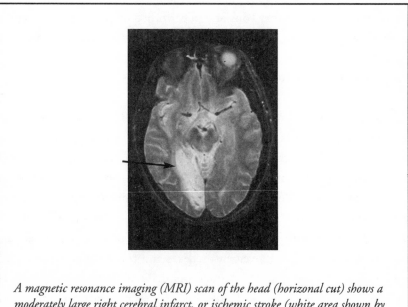

A magnetic resonance imaging (MRI) scan of the head (horizonal cut) shows a moderately large right cerebral infarct, or ischemic stroke (white area shown by arrow), in the posterior region several days after onset.

Imaging Tests

Since it may take some time for the damage caused by stroke to appear physically, your doctor may order imaging tests in the days following your stroke to assess the extent of the damage in the brain and to monitor your progress. These tests may include CT scans, magnetic resonance imaging (MRI), magnetic resonance angiography (MRA), and ultrasound. You are most likely to undergo your initial CT or MRI scan soon after you arrive; either or both of these tests may be repeated after that. Ischemic stroke is most visible on a CT scan from the third to tenth day after the stroke occurred. Hemorrhagic stroke is most visible on CT within the first seven to ten days. MRI can detect small infarcts that CT cannot, as well as infarcts in the back part of the brain. It can also be used to distinguish ischemic stroke from hemorrhagic stroke for several weeks after the event occurred, which makes it valuable in diagnosing and assessing patients who do not report to the hospital immediately after experiencing symptoms. MRA, a variation of MRI that provides a picture of blood vessels, may be used to detect and locate the intracranial aneurysm or vascular malformation at the root of hemorrhagic stroke. It can also be used to evaluate the carotid arteries and detect blockages there. Ultrasound (or duplex scanners, which incorporate ultrasound technology) may be used to detect blockages in the carotid arteries. Either of these imaging procedures may be used to help determine whether surgical intervention is necessary and may be repeated to determine if a treatment has improved blood flow through the arteries. Another type of test that may be used to detect blockages in the carotid arteries is ocular pneumoplethysmography, or OPG, which measures the systolic blood pressure in the ophthalmic arteries, which supply blood to the eye. These arteries branch off from the carotid arteries.

Cerebral Arteriography

This test, which I explain in chapter 6, is a more definitive but also more invasive way to evaluate the blood vessels and circulation. It can be performed on the blood vessels within the skull and outside it and can detect blockages, narrowing, and blood vessel damage. It can be used to estimate the degree of narrowing in an artery and to study aneurysms and arteriovenous malformations. It is the gold standard for determining blood flow and detecting arterial blockages. Its results are the most precise. Since the proce-

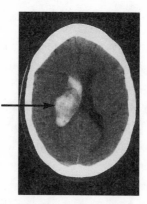

A. A computed tomography (CT) scan of the head (horizontal cut) indicates bleeding, or hemorrhage (white area shown by arrow), that originated in the right basal ganglia area of the brain.

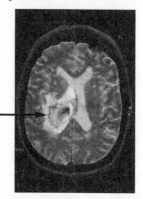

B. A magnetic resonance imaging (MRI) scan (horizontal cut) taken ten days after the CT scan shows the typical evolving appearance of hemorrhage over time (see arrow). This type of hemorrhage is typically caused by chronic hypertension.

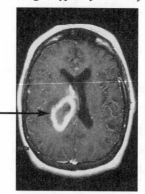

C. Another type of MRI (horizontal cut), taken at the same time as the previous one, also shows the evolution of the hemorrhage (see arrow).

dure does carry some risk, it is generally not used unless the result is necessary to determine a specific course of therapy. You might undergo this procedure, for example, if your doctor suspects that your stroke has been caused by a blockage in one of the smaller arteries of the head, by a small intracranial aneurysm, or by arteritis or arterial dissection (a situation in which the inner lining of the artery folds in on itself).

Blood Tests

Many of the blood tests I mention in chapter 6 are administered or repeated in the days following stroke. Blood tests that measure clotting factors and blood viscosity may be performed before a medication is prescribed or repeated some days later to determine if a medication is having the desired effect. Your doctor may use the results of other blood tests to diagnose blood conditions that may be an underlying cause of stroke, to aid in the diagnosis of atherosclerosis or diabetes, or to diagnose or rule out infection.

Cardiac Monitoring

Because many ischemic strokes are caused by cardiac problems, if you have had an ischemic stroke, you will likely undergo cardiovascular monitoring in the days following your stroke. This may include regular or possibly continuous electrocardiography to monitor your heart's electrical activity and rhythm, and echocardiography, which enables your doctor to visualize your heart, including clots and possible sources of clots. It can also assess heart function.

Brain Monitoring

In some cases, your doctor may need additional information and order an electroencephalogram, or EEG. This test measures the electrical activity in the brain. The test can be used to diagnose stroke in a patient who is comatose, although it is not ideal for determining what type of stroke is present. It can also be used to evaluate seizures that may accompany or follow stroke. Also of occasional value are two imaging tests that monitor brain metabolism. Positron emission tomography (PET) and single photon emission computed tomography (SPECT) create computer-generated X-ray images of the brain that track harmless radioactive isotopes that are injected or inhaled in the body. These tests, which can show how the brain is using

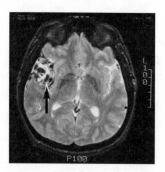

A. A magnetic resonance imaging (MRI) scan of the head (horizontal cut) indicates an arteriovenous malformation in the right temporal region of the brain (see arrow).

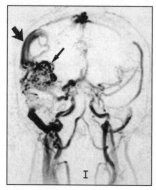

B. Magnetic resonance angiography (MRA) of the head (front view) shows the blood vessels, including an arteriovenous malformation (see small arrow), multiple enlarged, or dilated, feeding vessels from the right internal carotid artery, and a large draining vein (see large arrow).

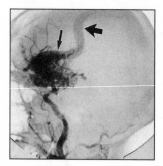

C. A cerebral arteriogram (side view) with dye injected into the common carotid artery showing the same arteriovenous malformation as in A and B (see small arrow) and an enlarged vein (see large arrow) draining blood for the malformation.

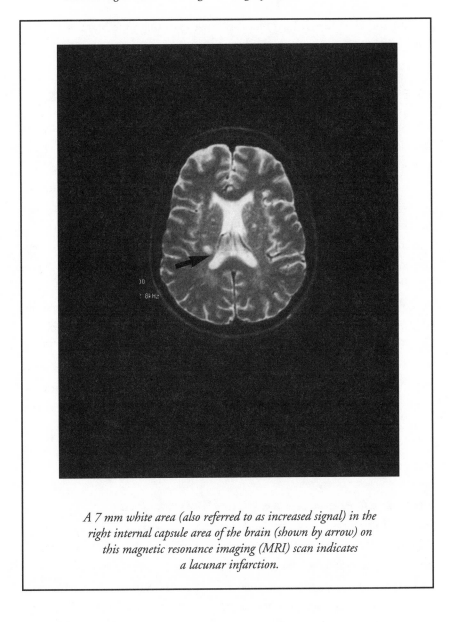

*A 7 mm white area (also referred to as increased signal) in the
right internal capsule area of the brain (shown by arrow) on
this magnetic resonance imaging (MRI) scan indicates
a lacunar infarction.*

oxygen and glucose and how blood is flowing through the brain, are generally available only at large medical centers.

PREVENTING AND ADDRESSING COMPLICATIONS

Damage assessment is only one part of continuing stroke treatment. Another key element is preventing complications—or addressing them if they occur. I touch on this briefly in chapter 6 during my discussion of subarachnoid hemorrhage. Preventing complications is a primary part of acute treatment for subarachnoid hemorrhage because the risk of complications is high during the first twenty-four hours. That risk doesn't simply disappear overnight, and it exists for other types of stroke as well. For example, about 20 percent of people who have survived an ischemic stroke die within thirty days, often from such complications as pneumonia, cardiac disorders, pulmonary embolism, and sepsis (blood poisoning). Not all complications of stroke are life-threatening, but many can cause a person's overall condition to deteriorate. Even minor complications can delay healing and rehabilitation. That's why continuing stroke care includes monitoring for complications and treating them as they arise. You have enough to worry about dealing with the consequences of your stroke. You don't need the additional physical and emotional stress of complicating conditions to retard your recovery.

Here's a rundown of the potential complications of stroke and how we address them:

Increased Pressure and Cerebral Swelling

Increased intracranial pressure and swelling, or edema, common complications of hemorrhagic stroke, also occur in some instances of ischemic stroke, notably those in which a large area of the brain has been deprived of blood and oxygen. The underlying causes of these complications differ depending on stroke type, but they produce similar symptoms. They are usually recognized during a physical examination. They often cause a decreased level of consciousness, produce swelling in the back of the eyes that is visible during an ophthalmic examination, and may affect the ability to move the eye or eyes outward. To reduce the swelling and relieve pressure, a doctor will likely place you on bed rest, elevate the head of your bed, and restrict fluids; he or she may prescribe steroids (particularly after a hemorrhagic stroke),

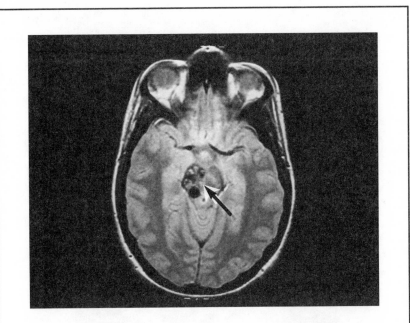

A.   A magnetic resonance imaging (MRI) scan of the head (horizontal cut) shows a small, relatively unusual blood vessel malformation called a cavernous hemiangioma involving the brain stem (see arrow).

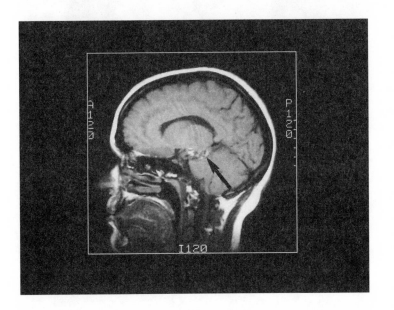

B.   An MRI sagittal image (cut down the middle of the head from front to back) shows the same cavernous malformation (see arrow).

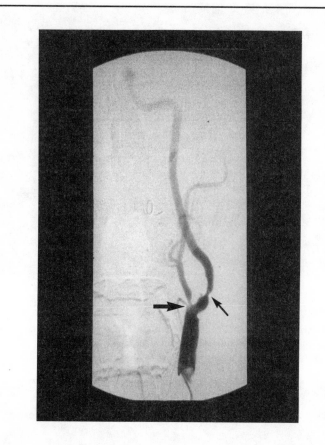

A cerebral arteriogram with dye injected into the common carotid artery shows a 70 percent narrowing, or stenosis, of the internal carotid artery (small arrow) and a 50 percent narrowing of the external carotid artery (large arrow).

which reduce inflammation and swelling, or such drugs as mannitol, glycerol, or diuretics, which cause the body to eliminate fluid. If these medications do not have the desired effect or the condition continues to worsen, surgery to relieve the pressure is a possibility.

Deep Vein Thrombosis and Pulmonary Embolism

These potentially life-threatening complications develop largely because stroke leaves many of its victims bedridden, which restricts circulation. In deep vein thrombosis, a clot, or *thrombus,* develops in one of the deep veins of the body, often those of the leg. This causes swelling, pain, tenderness, and skin discoloration. The primary danger in deep vein thrombosis, which occurs in up to 10 percent of patients with ischemic stroke, is that the clot will move toward the lungs, where it may block a major branch of the pulmonary artery. This is known as *pulmonary embolism.* Pulmonary embolism causes sudden chest pain, shock, and sudden shortness of breath. It can kill. In fact, it is fatal about 25 percent of the time.

Since pulmonary embolism accounts for 10 percent of deaths among patients who have had ischemic stroke, doctors generally take precautions to prevent and treat deep vein thrombosis—and watch carefully for the development of pulmonary embolism.

If you've had a stroke and are able to walk or move around, you will be advised to do so. Follow that advice. Don't be tempted—as some of my patients have been—to give in to the standard thinking that you are sick, so you must stay in bed. This is one instance in which that thinking can be deadly. If you've had a stroke and are bedridden, your doctor may order the foot of your bed to be elevated and ask you to wear compression stockings. If your stroke was ischemic, your doctor may also prescribe a low dose of the anticoagulant heparin to prevent the development of deep vein thrombosis.

If you do develop the condition, you will be given a higher dose of heparin and will likely be asked regularly if you're experiencing chest pain or breathing difficulties. If your doctor suspects that a pulmonary embolism has developed, you will be given heparin and may be asked to undergo several diagnostic tests, including a chest X ray, electrocardiogram, and arterial blood gas studies. If you are diagnosed with pulmonary embolism, anticoagulant therapy will likely continue for an extended time.

Pulmonary embolism after hemorrhagic stroke is much more difficult to treat. Anticoagulants, as you know, can cause hemorrhage, particularly in people who are prone to hemorrhage. And people who have had a hemorrhagic stroke definitely qualify. Our standard treatment could be worse than the original condition. Sometimes the best solution is a surgical procedure in which a vena cava umbrella (a filter) is installed in the vena cava, the main vein returning blood to the heart. This may filter out blood clots that originate in the legs.

Pneumonia

Nearly one-third of ischemic stroke patients develop pneumonia, which can be life-threatening. This lung inflammation, which can be caused by bacteria, viruses, or fungi, generally results in high fever, chest pain, and cough and can affect breathing. It is often complicated by sepsis (blood poisoning). To prevent pneumonia, you may be instructed to begin to move as early as possible and to practice deep breathing exercises. Because one form of pneumonia, aspiration pneumonia, develops as the result of taking vomit or other foreign material into the lungs, your ability to swallow may be tested before you are allowed to eat normal food. If you develop pneumonia, you will likely be given antibiotics to kill the bacteria that are causing it or to prevent a secondary bacterial infection.

Cardiovascular Complications

The cardiovascular and cerebrovascular systems are connected and interrelated. Just as cardiovascular problems can cause ischemic stroke, ischemic stroke can trigger cardiovascular complications. Among the most common are arrhythmias, or abnormal heart rhythms, and damage to the myocardium, or heart muscle. These problems are generally detected during the routine cardiovascular monitoring that occurs after stroke. They are usually treated with medications, and efforts are made to find and treat the underlying cause of the problem.

Seizures

Although seizures are more common with intracerebral hemorrhage, these sudden involuntary episodes occur in only about 10 percent of patients with ischemic stroke, generally within the first year after the stroke. They are generally treated with anticonvulsant medications.

Electrolyte Imbalances

Electrolyte imbalances—unbalanced quantities of such substances as sodium and potassium that conduct electrical current and are essential to a number of body processes—are relatively common among people who have had a subarachnoid hemorrhage and can occur as complications of other stroke types. The most common of these imbalances is sodium depletion, which affects about one-third of patients within two to ten days after subarachnoid hemorrhage. In the extreme, sodium depletion can affect consciousness, causing seizures and coma. Doctors focus their attention on finding the cause of the depletion, which varies from patient to patient. In some cases, the problem is caused by giving the patient too much fluid; in others, it is caused by a disease or condition that depletes the body of sodium; still others result from an overabundance of antidiuretic hormone. Treatment, obviously, involves slowly restoring sodium to the body and addressing the underlying problem.

Other electrolytes can also be depleted or present in excessively high levels. These include potassium, calcium, magnesium, and chloride.

Urinary Tract Infection

Ischemic stroke can affect your ability to control your bladder, causing incontinence or the opposite, urine retention. As a result, urinary tract infection is a potential complication. This, in turn, can often be complicated by sepsis (blood poisoning), which can be fatal. Your doctor will do what he or she can to help prevent you from developing one of these infections. Although you may need a catheter to help you urinate, catheters that stay in place for long periods of time can increase the risk of urinary tract infection. For this reason, your doctor may recommend frequent, temporary catheterization. Medications, too, may help address the underlying problems that can lead to urinary tract infection. Antibiotics are used to treat infection when it does occur.

Decubitus Ulcers (Bedsores)

Bedsores, like deep vein thrombosis and pulmonary embolism, are largely the result of being bedridden. These sores, known medically as decubitus ulcers, result from the continuous pressure placed on the skin covering such bony areas as the hips and shoulders when a person is bedridden. The pressure impedes the flow of blood and kills tissue, resulting in a sore or wound. Bedsores themselves generally are minor irritations. They are treated by cleaning the area and applying a topical medication. If they become infected, however, they can be life-threatening. Fortunately, many bedsores can be prevented. Air mattresses and tight bed sheets can help reduce pressure overall; keeping skin clean and dry can prevent irritation and infection; and adjusting position every few hours can reduce pressure on specific areas.

In addition to these complications, which are common to all forms of stroke, your doctor will continue his or her attempts to prevent and/or treat those complications of subarachnoid hemorrhage I discuss in chapter 6: rebleeding, vasospasm, and hydrocephalus.

TREATING UNDERLYING CAUSES AND PREVENTING RECURRENT STROKE

By this point, you know that stroke is nearly always the result of one or more underlying diseases or conditions. These are not always readily identifiable, although they are identified in the majority of cases. If we are not able to identify the underlying cause or causes, ongoing stroke treatment consists of conservative, general measures, for example, antiplatelet agents and continued diagnostic testing, if necessary. In most situations, the hallmark of continuing stroke treatment is addressing the underlying cause or causes of stroke. This serves the dual purpose of treating the underlying condition and reducing the risk of subsequent stroke. In fact, some of the treatments I discuss in this chapter are discussed in more detail in the stroke prevention chapters—4 and 5. This is no mistake. Stroke prevention and treatment are integrally related and, in some ways, one and the same. Approximately 10 percent of stroke survivors will have another stroke within a year, and the five-year rate of subsequent stroke is about 25 to 30 percent for ischemic stroke. If you've had a stroke, you are clearly at risk of having another, and secondary prevention should be a major goal of your treatment.

The number and types of treatments used in the aftermath of stroke are as numerous and varied as the conditions that cause stroke. The information I provide here should give you an overall understanding of the types of treatment that are available for each stroke subtype. The treatment your doctor chooses for you will depend on your overall health, the type and severity of your stroke, the underlying cause or causes of your stroke, and any other conditions you have that may affect your health, recovery, and risk.

Ischemic Stroke

Continuing treatment for ischemic stroke often involves such blood-thinning medications as anticoagulants and antiplatelet agents. It may also include medications to control high blood pressure and, depending on the cause of the stroke and your overall condition, surgery.

ATHEROSCLEROTIC ISCHEMIC STROKE

Atherosclerotic ischemic stroke is caused by atherosclerosis, a buildup of fatty deposits known as plaque on the insides of artery walls. This buildup narrows the arteries and attracts blood products, increasing the risk of clots and blockages. It can cause stroke if it appears in the arteries in the neck or any of the arteries or arterioles in the head that supply the brain. Treatment for this atherosclerotic ischemic stroke depends on several factors, including the location and extent of atherosclerotic buildup and the patient's overall health.

If atherosclerotic buildup narrows one or more of the carotid arteries by 70 percent or more and the patient is in generally good health, carotid endarterectomy is likely to be the treatment of choice, particularly if the initial ischemic stroke was minor and recent. This surgical procedure, which I detail in chapter 4, involves scraping the inner lining of the carotid artery to remove the built-up plaque. Its primary purpose is to prevent future stroke. Carotid endarterectomy may also be recommended if atherosclerosis narrows a carotid artery by 50 to 69 percent. The procedure is unlikely to be helpful if the carotid is narrowed by less than 50 percent.

In some situations, other high-tech interventions may be used. Angioplasty, a procedure in which a balloon is inflated inside an artery, is currently being investigated as a treatment for carotid artery blockage. It can also be used to open up another artery that supplies the brain, for example, one of the vertebral arteries. Artery-artery bypass surgery may be used in rare situations. These procedures are discussed in detail in chapter 4.

If there is a known complete blockage of the carotid artery, if atherosclerotic buildup does not meet the criteria for carotid endarterectomy, if angioplasty or artery-artery bypass are not options, if the blockage is in an area of the brain that is hard to access, or if the patient suffers from another condition that could make surgery unwise—kidney or heart problems or uncontrolled diabetes or hypertension—treatment may be medical. It could begin with heparin and be followed by warfarin, and finally, daily aspirin or another antiplatelet agent, or it could begin with warfarin. Those who cannot take anticoagulants will likely be treated with antiplatelet medications from the beginning.

In addition to surgical or medical treatment, I often recommend a very-low-saturated-fat, very-low-cholesterol diet, regular physical activity, stress reduction, and treatment for hypertension and high cholesterol, if these conditions are present. I discuss my dietary and lifestyle recommendations in chapter 5. If the patient is a smoker, I will advise him or her to quit. I discuss methods for smoking cessation in chapter 4.

CARDIOEMBOLIC ISCHEMIC STROKE

Cardioembolic stroke, as you may recall, is the type of ischemic stroke generally associated with blood clots that originate in the heart. These clots ultimately make their way to an artery that supplies blood to the brain, causing brain attack. The two primary sources of these clots are diseased, scarred, or replacement heart valves and conditions that affect other parts of the heart, including atrial fibrillation, sick sinus syndrome, recent heart attack, congestive heart failure, and cardiomyopathy.

Regardless of the source of the clot, cardioembolic stroke is generally treated with anticoagulant therapy, usually intravenous heparin, followed by warfarin, which can be given orally. Since it takes five or six days for warfarin treatment to become effective, the two drugs may be given simultaneously for a short period. These medications help thin the blood and prevent the formation of additional clots. Patients who cannot take anticoagulants may be given antiplatelet medications instead for the same reason.

If your doctor has determined what caused the clot to develop, you may also undergo treatment aimed at the underlying cause. If your stroke was caused by a clot that formed on one of your heart valves, for example, your treatment may also include surgery to repair or replace the damaged valve. If you have been diagnosed with sick sinus syndrome, your doctor may recommend installation of a pacemaker to restore a normal heart rhythm. Likewise, if you have recently been diagnosed with atrial fibrillation, your doctor may recommend cardioversion, or shock therapy, to restore the normal heart rhythm. Chronic atrial fibrillation is generally treated with long-term anticoagulant therapy. If congestive heart failure or cardiomyopathy is the source of the problem, your treatment could also include digitalis, diuretics, bed rest, and restriction of sodium and fluids. Regardless of your underlying condition, you will likely undergo regular cardiac monitoring with echocardiography to monitor your progress. For an in-depth discussion of the treatment of various cardiac conditions, see chapter 4.

LACUNAR STROKE

Lacunar stroke is generally caused by chronic high blood pressure. Blood pressure should be reduced, but gradually. Major, rapid drops in blood pressure can cause infarction. Thus, blood pressure must be reduced in a slow and controlled way. As you know, numerous medications are available to reduce high blood pressure. I describe the various types of antihypertensives in detail in chapter 4. The doctor will tailor his or her selection of medications to the patient's individual needs. In addition to medication, the doctor will likely recommend a low-fat, low-cholesterol diet, regular physical activity, and smoking cessation. In some cases, he or she might also recommend antiplatelet therapy, although this treatment is of unproven benefit for lacunar stroke. Treatment for lacunar stroke seldom includes anticoagulants, which carry more potential for risk.

OTHER

The other category, as its name implies, is a catchall category for ischemic strokes caused by conditions that simply don't fit into the more common categories of ischemic stroke. These include blood disorders that increase blood's likelihood to clot, infections, and other conditions. Needless to say, the treatments for strokes that fall into this category are numerous. I can give you a general idea of the types of treatments that may be recommended.

Noninfectious arteritis, vascular inflammation related to any of a number of conditions, including lupus, may be treated with steroids to reduce the inflammation and sometimes other medications to treat the underlying condition. Infectious arteritis and the underlying bacterial infections that cause it, including endocarditis and syphilis, are generally treated with antibiotics. Fungal infections like aspergillosis are treated with antifungal medications, while viral infections like herpes zoster are treated with antiviral agents. Such blood diseases as thrombocythemia and antiphospholipid antibody syndromes, in which antibodies in the blood affect clotting, may be treated with anticoagulants or antiplatelet agents. Treatment of polycythemia may also involve phlebotomy (removal of blood); treatment of thrombocythemia may involve plateletpheresis (removal of platelets); and treatment for thrombocytopenic purpura may involve plasmapheresis (removal of plasma from the blood). Sickle-cell disease may be treated with red blood cell transfusions and lifestyle changes designed to maintain an adequate supply of oxygen in the blood. The choice of treatment depends on the underlying condition and the individual's overall health. I discuss the treatment of many of these conditions in more detail in chapter 4.

Hemorrhagic Stroke

The blood-thinning agents that play such a major role in the continuing treatment of ischemic stroke have no place in the treatment of hemorrhagic stroke, which is characterized by bleeding. Treatment for this less common type of stroke is more likely to involve other medications, surgery, blood pressure control, and monitoring for hemorrhagic complications.

SUBARACHNOID HEMORRHAGE

The most common cause of subarachnoid hemorrhage, or bleeding outside the brain, is the rupture of an intracranial aneurysm. You might think that once an aneurysm has ruptured little can be done to treat it. An aneurysm can actually rerupture, causing bleeding again. Along with preventing vasospasm, which I discuss in chapter 6, this is what continuing stroke treatment is designed to avoid. The most common and traditional treatment for a ruptured aneurysm is surgical clipping, which cuts the ballooning off from the blood supply. An alternate treatment involves placing coils in the aneurysm to cause it to clot off and separate itself from the circulation or perform another type of endovascular procedure to reduce the likelihood that the aneurysm will bleed again. The earlier these procedures (described in more detail in chapter 4) can be performed, the better, but not every patient is a candidate for immediate treatment. The severity of the hemorrhage and the patient's overall health and condition have an effect on the outcome and the choice of treatment. If surgery or coiling are not options, the doctor may recommend monitoring and general care, and possibly a procedure in the future if it becomes feasible.

Subarachnoid hemorrhage can also be caused by the rupture of a vascular malformation. These ruptures are generally managed conservatively at first to prevent the increase of intracranial pressure, then surgically removed, if possible, one or two weeks after the hemorrhage has occurred. Other treatment options include embolization to cut off feeding vessels, proton beam radiation, and gamma knife radiosurgery, a highly focused, three-dimensional beam of radiation guided by a computer to a precise target, for example, the nidus, or center, of a vascular malformation that is located in an inoperable area or otherwise cannot be removed. This causes the lining of the vascular walls to enlarge, which eventually closes the malformation, cutting it off from the circulation. This and other forms of radiation are less risky than surgery, but it does take from one to three years for the malformation to close off altogether. I discuss these techniques in more detail in chapter 4.

INTRACEREBRAL HEMORRHAGE

As with subarachnoid hemorrhage, treatment for intracerebral hemorrhage depends on the cause. Since the most common cause is chronic high blood pressure, antihypertensive medication is one of the mainstays of treatment. As with treatment for lacunar ischemic stroke, the choice of medication will depend on the individual. In addition, steroids, or drugs like mannitol and glycerol, or diuretics may be prescribed to reduce swelling in the brain. If a large amount of blood has pooled in the brain, surgery may be necessary to drain the pool, or hematoma. This procedure, known as evacuation, may also be performed to drain large hematomas in intracerebral hemorrhages caused by other factors. These factors include ruptured aneurysms and vascular malformations, which although most likely to cause subarachnoid hemorrhage, can also cause intracerebral hemorrhage. These ruptures are treated in the same manner as they are treated for subarachnoid hemorrhage. Intracerebral hemorrhages caused by disorders that promote bleeding or prevent clotting, thrombocytopenia and hemophilia for example, may be treated with transfusions of platelets or other blood components that help the blood clot. When anticoagulant therapy is the underlying cause, the component used is fresh frozen plasma, often in addition to vitamin K. These two treatments help reverse the effect of the medication.

REHABILITATION

Once the immediate danger is over and the underlying cause of stroke is addressed, we turn our attention to rehabilitation—the process in which you regain as much of your previous abilities as possible and learn to adapt to any remaining deficits. Needless to say, the type and amount of rehabilitation you receive depend on the type and extent of difficulties you have. Likewise, these factors play a major role in the extent to which you can be rehabilitated.

Sadly, stroke kills approximately 20 percent of its victims each year. It is also a leading cause of disability. More than 3 million of today's stroke survivors have some degree of disability. Approximately one-third of younger stroke survivors and approximately three-quarters of older stroke survivors are permanently impaired or disabled by stroke. Studies indicate that one-half to two-thirds of stroke survivors regain their independence, and up to 80 percent retain or regain their ability to walk. Likewise, approximately half of stroke survivors are able to return to work after their stroke. In this arena, younger people fare better than older people. About 80 percent of stroke survivors age thirty to thirty-nine are able to return to some type of job.

The range of disability and rehabilitation is virtually infinite. I've had patients who have completely recovered from serious deficits in a matter of minutes; I've had patients who have worked for months and never improved; and I've seen virtually everything in between. It's impossible to predict with certainty how far a person will progress, because so many variables are involved, including the type and extent of stroke damage, the patient's overall health, the quality of the rehabilitation team, the support of family and friends, and the patient's attitude.

A good rehabilitation team should be able to give you a realistic idea of what you can reasonably expect to accomplish and how long it will take. With a lot of work and the right attitude, you may be able to exceed the team's expectations, but it will be largely up to you to reach your goal.

To give you a general idea, the probability of improvement of movement in paralyzed limbs is best in the first few months after a stroke. It decreases significantly after six months and rarely continues for over a year or two. Recovery of arm movement is less likely to be complete than recovery of leg movement. What we call *functional recovery*—the lessening of disability that results from the combination of physical recovery and adaptation—can continue for a long time after you stop making physical improvement. In addition, speech, working skills, and steadiness can continue to improve for as long as two years or even more.

I want to stress that statistics are meaningless when it comes to individual cases. Like any adversity, recovering from stroke tests us and reveals us in sometimes surprising ways. The support of medical professionals and close family and friends is a vital part of the rehabilitation equation. The internal resources we may never have known we had can make the biggest difference.

Rebecca was a forty-five-year-old professional dancer. During rehearsal one day, she suffered a brain stem hemorrhage from a vascular malformation—unfortunately in a location we couldn't operate on without a high risk of killing her. This talented dancer was not only paralyzed on the left side of her body and face, she was also in danger of having her malformation rupture again.

Her treatment and recovery were arduous. Though she wasn't a candidate for conventional surgery, we were able to treat the malformation with gamma knife radiosurgery. As is commonly the case, she had a lot of swelling after the radiosurgical treatments, which required long courses of steroids over many months. The steroids caused her considerable weight gain, which is depressing for anyone, much less a dancer.

But Rebecca never lost sight of her goal, which was to dance again, and she never let herself become discouraged. She plunged tirelessly into physical rehabilitation, gradually recovering the full use of her limbs and facial muscles. It took her almost a full year of hard work, but she is now dancing professionally again. Though she herself acknowledges that she's lost a few steps from her physical prime, people who had seen her perform before her stroke believe that she's more expressive and eloquent a dancer than ever.

It is not my intent to detail all the particulars of rehabilitation. Other authors have devoted entire books to the subject, and I recommend some good references in the appendix to this book. My goal in this chapter is to outline a few basic principles that I have found are critical to the success of rehabilitation.

Assemble a Good Rehabilitation Team

Although you will ultimately do much of the work during rehabilitation, you need a good, competent team to direct and advise you—just as an athlete in training needs a top-notch coaching staff. This team is led by your neurologist, physiatrist (a doctor who specializes in physical medicine and rehabilitation), or other physician knowledgeable about stroke and stroke rehabilitation. Your team may also include rehabilitation nurses, a psychologist to help you deal with the emotional effects of stroke, and a social worker to help you and your family prepare your home. Depending on your needs, you may work with one or more of the following therapists: physical, occupational, and speech. The team leader, like a head coach, coordinates your care; the psychologist, social worker, and therapists each coach you in the aspects of rehabilitation in which they specialize.

Physical therapists evaluate your level of physical disability and help you work toward maintaining your remaining physical functions and recovering those you may have lost. These are the individuals who will work with you to keep your weakened or paralyzed limbs flexible and help you regain strength and movement, primarily with guided exercise and proper positioning of your limbs. They may help you learn how to move about in bed, then to sit, to stand, and to use a wheelchair independently. Ultimately, they may be able to help you relearn how to walk, alone or with the help of a walker or cane.

Occupational therapists teach patients how to adapt to everyday life. These are the individuals who will teach you how to sit up, stand up, and transfer from one place to another if one side of your body is paralyzed. They may help you relearn how to eat, dress, bathe, and perform other daily activities, using exercises and adaptive equipment.

Speech-language pathologists (speech therapists) diagnose your communication disabilities and help you regain your ability to communicate if it has been lost. They may help you exercise and retrain affected speech muscles or compensate for other communication deficits by using your skills. For example, they may encourage you to write or use gestures if you cannot speak. Or they may introduce computers or other communication devices.

You may or may not need these various therapists on your team. It depends on your individual needs. (At Mayo Clinic, about half of all patients who survive ischemic stroke for one week are good candidates to benefit from physical therapy, about 40 percent from occupational therapy, and about 15 percent from speech therapy.) I cannot emphasize enough how important it is to have a rehabilitation team who address all of your various needs in a competent, complementary fashion. These are the individuals who will help you set reasonable goals and guide you as you work toward those goals. No matter how determined and dedicated you are, you need this direction. Chances are, it's been a long time since you learned to walk, talk, and take care of yourself. Even then, you did it with the help of your family. Your family is still an important factor: Family members can help you with your exercises and offer needed emotional support, but you need professional guidance as well.

Set Clear, Reasonable Goals

Your rehabilitation team will help you set reasonable goals for rehabilitation. Use these to guide you. Although it's fine to have a larger goal in mind for the future and to work toward that larger goal, be sure to tackle the smaller goals first. If you are unable to walk, for example, walking may be your ultimate, long-term goal. Chances are, you will need to work progressively toward that goal, first learning to stand, then learning to walk with adaptive equipment before you can amble on your own. Setting clear, reasonable goals makes achieving them easier, gives you a feeling of success, and helps you avoid becoming discouraged.

Think about what you want to accomplish. Talk your goals over with members of your rehabilitation team to see if they think the goals are reasonable. Discuss them with your family. They may have suggestions, and you may be able to enlist their help in working toward your goals. Remember: The ultimate decision rests with you. It is you who will resolve what to accomplish, and you who will accomplish it.

Use Your Affected Parts

You know the old saying, "Use it or lose it." Well, it could have been written with stroke rehabilitation in mind. Although your stroke may have made you temporarily unable to use certain abilities the way you were able, if you don't attempt to use them, you may lose them permanently. Although there is no guarantee that exercise will help you regain muscle function, I can guarantee that you will not regain muscle function if you don't do the range-of-motion and strength-training exercises designed for that purpose and instead let muscles go idle. Likewise, if stroke has affected your cognitive function, you need to "exercise" your mind and use your mental function.

If you're suffering from aphasia, the loss of communication skills I describe in chapter 2, it's very easy to get discouraged, particularly if you are an articulate, quick-minded person who is used to having full command of your communication skills. In many cases, this discouragement causes patients to avoid using their communication skills altogether, but this is the wrong tack to take. You need to work your mind and speech organs in order to regain your communication skills.

If there is a physical problem, for example, if stroke has affected your control of the muscles needed to speak, the speech therapist may concentrate on physical exercise and position. He or she may work with you to strengthen and tone the affected muscles, physically position your lips and tongue in the proper place for speech, and help you breathe properly. If you have difficulty understanding spoken words, for example, the therapist may speak the names of certain objects and ask you to point to them, or to pictures of them. Later, you may progress to executing simple commands, such as "Pick up the radio," or "Point to the spoon," or to answering yes or no questions about a series of pictures. If you have difficulties with printed language, your therapist may ask you to read single words, match words to pictures, arrange words into phrases, execute printed commands, or read short paragraphs. If you have trouble speaking, your speech therapist may ask you to answer simple yes or no questions, then encourage you to engage in longer, more complicated conversation. As you can see, these tasks are usually progressive, as are the steps in learning to use language for the first time. Like learning anything for the first time, relearning takes repetition and practice.

The same holds true for limb paralysis. It can be very discouraging to try and fail time after time. That discouragement can cause you to avoid working your muscles and lead you to a kind of learned helplessness that can lessen your chances of recovery. If you faithfully practice range-of-motion exercises and exercises to strengthen your muscles, then progress to exercises in balance, you are likely to see progress eventually.

This is not simply a give-it-your-best recommendation designed to get you to do "something." It has scientific merit. Stroke affects the brain's circuitry, causing breaks in the electrical pathways through which your functions are controlled. Your brain contains billions of neurons, or nerve cells. Extensions of these cells known as dendrites receive electrical impulses sent from the axons of other nerve cells. Axons are extensions of the nerve cells that conduct electrical impulses from the cell. This is how your brain sends messages. As you may recall from chapter 2, stroke kills or damages neurons in the area of the brain where it occurs. Neurons that have died cannot be replaced, but damaged neurons may be revived through use. Attempts to perform a function affected by the death of certain neurons may also spark the growth of axons and dendrites in other neurons to complete the circuit. Your best way to reconnect circuits interrupted by stroke—or to reroute them to other brain pathways—is to try to use them—in other words, to do what you are having difficulty doing.

Maintain a Positive Outlook

Although the effects of stroke can be downright depressing and progress can be slow, try not to get discouraged. It's counterproductive. It's natural to go through anger, depression, disbelief, and grief, but a continually negative attitude can hinder or retard your recovery. Research indicates, for example, that depression can have a negative impact on your physical health. It's been linked to an increased risk of hypertension and heart disease. A colleague of mine in the psychiatric department at Mayo Clinic has recently published findings of a study that indicated that being a pessimist—specifically explaining life events in a negative way—increases the risk of an early death.

Your attitude is absolutely crucial to your physical health and to the success of your rehabilitation. If you have a pessimistic outlook, you will approach rehabilitation passively, believing that what you do won't make a difference. This can become a self-fulfilling prophecy. On the other hand, if you adopt a positive outlook, you will be more likely to work toward your goals, which means you will be more likely to achieve them. I've seen first-hand how attitude can affect recovery and rehabilitation progress for better and worse.

Sandra's recovery is a good case in point. The fifty-year-old business executive came to see me months after an ischemic stroke had left her with serious communication deficits. Normally quick, bright, and articulate, she was also a public speaker—an important part of her professional identity. She used to travel and speak at conferences around the country where she was a tireless public voice for her company. Now she struggled to find words and complete sentences. She was tremendously frustrated and embarrassed in public.

Sandra came to me for advice on what she could do to regain her speech abilities and to prevent a future stroke. I advised her to change her diet and to begin an exercise program. I also referred her to one of my colleagues in the speech pathology department. He designed a therapy program for her that encouraged her to continue to use her intellect and speech, even though it was difficult and discouraging for her. As I tracked her progress, I was impressed by Sandra's mix of pragmatism and tenacity. She set monthly goals for herself and worked doggedly toward them. She also took the practical steps of redesigning her work routine to adapt to her deficits and rehabilitation. She temporarily stopped public speaking and took on more writing projects, but she kept working at recovering every nuance of speech.

It took her about two years to fully recover her language ability. Ultimately, she returned to her very intellectually demanding job, and now does even more public speaking than before. She talks proudly about her rehabilitation and prizes the hard-won lessons she's learned about herself.

Michelle is another example of the power of a positive perspective. The forty-seven-year-old administrative assistant suffered a warning leak from an intracranial aneurysm and went to her local emergency room. The doctors frankly misdiagnosed her sudden, sharp headache, stiff neck, and nausea as a severe tension headache. They prescribed analgesics, and three days later, she suffered a subarachnoid hemorrhage.

By the time she came to see us, she was in a coma. She recovered somewhat over the next few days, although she had visual disturbances and difficulty speaking or writing, and we clipped her aneurysm. Another patient might have become embittered over the misdiagnosis she received when she went to the emergency room. Michelle simply felt thankful to be alive. Although she still had some language deficits after the surgery, she remained positive throughout her rehabilitation, which continued to bear fruit.

Within six months of her surgery, Michelle was fully recovered and she was able to resume all her normal activities.

Your attitude is one aspect of your recovery over which you have control. Do whatever you can to adopt a positive attitude. Know that you may become discouraged, and plan on things you can do to overcome your discouragement. Find new ways to be useful, new ways to help others. Decide what you want to do in life and what you want to get out of it, and start working toward that goal. Realize that your efforts to overcome your disability can be a real inspiration to those around you. Since what you project to others is often reflected back to you, you may reap additional benefits from your positive outlook.

I've related some remarkable stories of full recovery, but I want to stress that recovering specific faculties isn't the only meaningful measure of rehabilitation. What counts most is recovering your ability to enjoy life—the activities that give you pleasure and the company of people who make you happy.

Margaret was one of my favorite patients and a continual inspiration to me. At age sixty, she was afflicted with a rare form of brain artery inflammation that is often fatal. In Margaret's case, we were able to control the inflammation, but not its recurrence. During the next twenty years, she would suffer from painful and frightening flare-ups that we had to treat and control. She had to spend a good deal of time in the hospital, and we had to treat her with powerful medications, ranging from steroids to antimetabolic drugs ordinarily used in cancer treatment.

Through it all, Margaret was unfailingly positive. Instead of focusing on her suffering, she always talked about how grateful she was to be alive, how lucky she was to still have her husband and to be enjoying her grandchildren. In between her bouts of inflammation, she cultivated her chief pleasures in life: gardening and writing. Over the years, she shared her poetry and stories with me, which I took as a great gift. And she managed to share her caring personality with countless patients wherever she encountered them. No matter how much physical distress she was in, it never blinded her to the suffering of others. No matter how frightening an episode she faced, she never lost sight of everything she still treasured about living.

I count Margaret as one of my best teachers. I've learned so much from her about the importance of seizing life in the midst of disease, about the power of the spirit to overcome the physical infirmities that inevitably await us all. Margaret has taught me the true meaning of rehabilitation, which literally means "to restore." I've learned from her that rehabilitation is less about restoring the body than about restoring the soul, less about restoring our neural pathways than it is about restoring the connection to the life force within us.

8

On the Horizon: The Future of Stroke Risk Assessment, Prevention, and Treatment

Mike and Carol Jones, both twenty-nine, have appointments for themselves and their five-year-old daughter, Kathy, at the stroke prevention clinic. Mike is due for a routine checkup. He'll have his blood pressure and cholesterol levels checked and get a refill of the angiotensin II inhibitor he's been taking to stave off atrial fibrillation, congestive heart failure, atherosclerosis, and hypertension. Carol will visit the clinic for the first time. She scheduled the appointment after learning that she has a genetic predisposition to develop atherosclerosis. She will tell the doctor about her personal and family medical history and be physically examined. She will also undergo blood tests, including tests to identify markers of inflammation or inflammatory instability and subtle clotting changes that may place her at increased stroke risk, and echocardiography, an ultrasound test of the heart, to measure various physiological markers, including the volume of her left atrium. The doctor will use the results of these tests—along with information obtained during the examination and from her medical history—to determine whether Carol has any risk factors for stroke or if she, like Mike, is at risk of developing conditions that may increase her stroke risk. The couple scheduled Kathy for genetic screening after learning the results of Carol's genetic test. Kathy's blood will be drawn and analyzed to determine if she has genetic markers for several stroke risk factors, including the marker for atherosclerosis that Carol has. The results of the tests will enable the doctor to work with Mike and Carol to develop an appropriate stroke prevention plan for Kathy—to get her started on prevention early in life.

Although this scenario is futuristic, it is not unrealistic. In the future, stroke prevention centers will largely replace stroke treatment centers. I see a major shift in our focus—from reaction to preemptive action, from treatment to prevention, from dealing with endpoints to dealing with beginnings. The whole paradigm will shift to younger individuals. We will be able to do a better job of ridding the world of stroke and many of its underlying conditions.

Research is moving at a rapid pace. Each new risk factor we uncover, each new assessment tool we develop gives us a better picture of stroke and a clearer idea of how to prevent and treat it. We now have, for the first time, the means of predicting a person's stroke risk and tailoring preventive efforts to those specific risks. This alone is a significant development. In the next five to ten years, there is good reason to believe that we'll be able to go beyond simply identifying a person's risk factors and taking steps to reduce or eliminate them to predicting and even preventing their development. Some of these tools, a healthy diet, exercise, and stress reduction for example, are already in place, and more appear to be on the horizon.

This is clearly good news if you are at low risk of stroke. You may be able to put the proverbial cart before the horse, preventing some stroke risk factors as a way to prevent stroke. Those at low risk are not the only ones who will benefit from these advances. As research continues into the mechanics and causes of stroke, we will gain a better understanding of the role each risk factor plays. We may also uncover additional risk factors. These discoveries will enable us to tailor our preventive efforts further. Even though prevention will become our primary focus, we won't leave behind those who actually suffer strokes. In fact, stroke sufferers should see some of the most noticeable and dramatic improvements. The advances that have been made in treating stroke in the past decade have been extremely encouraging. We will continue to see improvement in everything from diagnosis to rehabilitation. Ultimately, the number of people who survive stroke and walk away without permanent disability will increase, and stroke will cease to be the powerful nemesis it now is.

RISK FACTORS

Risk factor identification—now the first step in prevention—will continue to play an important role. As research into the underlying causes and mechanics of stroke continues, we will obtain definitive answers about the role of such "conflicting" risk factors as estrogen, alcohol, cholesterol levels, depression, and stress.

In addition to refining information about risk factors we have already identified, we may identify new risk factors. Already, preliminary evidence indicates that chronic inflammation may be a risk factor for atherosclerosis and, subsequently, for ischemic stroke. If this proves to be the case, we may be able to use such markers of inflammation as C-reactive protein and elevated levels of certain white blood cells to identify the presence of chronic inflammation and determine who may be likely to develop atherosclerosis. Persistent inflammation with the bacterium *Chlamydia pneumoniae* has also been linked to the development of atherosclerosis. Blood tests can identify the presence of this bacterium. High blood levels of homocysteine, a naturally occurring amino acid, have also been linked in epidemiological studies to an increased risk of ischemic heart disease and ischemic stroke.

Researchers are also looking into genetic markers that may help identify people at risk for stroke. Studies of intracranial aneurysms, for example, are trying to identify and characterize the molecular genetic basis for predispositions to their development and rupture. We know that many people develop aneurysms that never rupture, and that people who have had an aneurysm rupture are more likely to have other aneurysms rupture. We are trying to determine whether the predisposition to develop aneurysms or the predisposition for rupture has a genetic component and whether that component can be easily identified.

In what may be one of the most exciting developments, the cardiology and cerebrovascular neurology divisions at Mayo Clinic have identified a marker we believe may be used to predict the development of atrial fibrillation, congestive heart failure, atherosclerosis, and possibly hypertension. We believe that these conditions may be related to—or even caused by—dysfunction of the endothelium, the layer of cells that lines the heart, blood vessels, and other body cavities, as well as diastolic dysfunction, dysfunction during the part of heartbeat when the heart is relaxed. Diastolic dysfunction, which is related to aging, hypertension, and other stresses to the cardiovascular and endothelial systems, causes the heart and blood vessels to become less elastic. In its early stages, it also causes the left atrium, or upper chamber of the heart, to enlarge. These changes have also been associated with increased coagulation or increased clotting and with various other bio-chemical abnormalities. If diastolic and endothelial dysfunction are indeed reliable precursors of atrial fibrillation, congestive heart failure, hyperten-sion, and atherosclerosis, we could measure the left atrial volume to deter-mine if patients are at risk of developing these stroke risk factors. We are currently investigating how good a good predictor of risk this measurement is, and preliminary results look very promising. This could have a rapid impact on risk factor assessment and prevention. It also has implications for preventive treatment, which I discuss below.

PREVENTION

New information about risk factors, obviously, will translate into new and more precise methods of prevention.

Risk Factor Prevention

As I mention in the previous section, there is reason to believe that various parameters that may be connected to an underlying endothelial dysfunc-tion, including enlarged left atrial volume, can predict the development of certain stroke risk factors. If this hypothesis is correct, shifting the focus of treatment to the underlying dysfunction could prevent these conditions from developing. A lot of theoretical evidence and some anecdotal evidence suggests that certain antihypertensive drugs, notably angiotensin II inhib-itors and, to a lesser extent, ACE inhibitors and beta-blockers, may be an effective treatment for this endothelial and diastolic dysfunction. Definitive evidence will need to await the results of large, randomized trials.

The concept of vascular protection is not without some precedent. Sev-eral recent studies have found that ACE inhibitors offer protection against cardiovascular disease and stroke even in people who do not require treat-ment for hypertension. In one major study, the use of the ACE inhibitor ramipril (Altace) reduced the combined risk of heart attack, stroke, and death from cardiovascular causes by 22 percent. It also reduced the risk of heart failure, cardiac arrest, and worsening angina.

These studies examined the effects of ACE inhibitors in a broad group of people and looked only at broad endpoints. We hope to take these findings to the next level. By targeting a specific group of at-risk people for treatment with angiotensin II inhibitors, ACE inhibitors, or beta-blockers, we may be able to reduce the risk of ischemic stroke by half or more. Other medical therapies could be more specifically targeted to reducing inflammatory instability or oxidative stress in the cardiovascular system and normalizing the balance between competing factors that promote and inhibit blood clotting.

Genetics could offer another path toward risk factor prevention. Once genetic markers are identified, it may be possible to screen people to find out whether they are at increased risk of developing certain risk factors. This could enable medical professionals and patients to take whatever actions they can to prevent those risk factors from developing. Eventually, genetic predispositions may be treatable with gene therapy. Currently in its experimental stages, gene therapy could be used to change a gene that predisposes a person to a specific risk factor. Gene therapy has also been advocated as a potential therapeutic treatment for stroke. Others have pointed to a number of ethical and biological hazards. These concerns, coupled with the fact that the genes in question have not yet been fully identified and the therapy techniques have not been perfected, mean that it will be at least some time before gene therapy plays a major role in stroke prevention.

Prevention Tool Improvement

The medications and interventional techniques we use to treat stroke risk factors and prevent stroke will continue to improve. New medications are constantly being developed, including new brands and classes of blood pressure medications, medications to lower cholesterol and triglycerides, and medications to treat diabetes mellitus. Several new antiplatelet agents have come on the market in recent years, and more are likely to be approved in the future. In addition, researchers and practitioners are experimenting with various combinations of agents to see if they increase effectiveness. These new medications will offer additional ammunition against the various conditions that increase stroke risk. Some may be major breakthroughs; most will likely offer a slight improvement in treatment or an alternative for patients who cannot take a similar drug.

Interventional procedures, too, will improve. In recent years, we have greatly refined our understanding of when carotid endarterectomy should be performed, and we should soon know more about carotid angioplasty. As I mention in chapter 4, this procedure is being used as a stroke preventive in some medical centers, but carotid angioplasty has not been widely studied or compared with carotid endarterectomy. Research is now under way to determine when carotid angioplasty is appropriate and when it is preferable to carotid endarterectomy. Researchers are also looking at whether this balloon procedure should be performed by itself or in conjunction with stenting (placing an object in the artery), to prevent atherosclerotic plaque from building up again at the same site.

Likewise, the endovascular procedures being used to prevent intracranial aneurysms and vascular malformations from rupturing are still being developed and refined. Technological advances in this area are ongoing. A scant ten years ago, balloons were the cutting edge of endovascular treatment for unruptured intracranial aneurysms. They've since been replaced by metallic coils, which are placed inside the aneurysm in most cases to isolate the aneurysm from the circulation. Several technical developments have occurred relevant to endovascular coiling techniques in the last five years.

DIAGNOSIS AND ASSESSMENT

Diagnostic technology is constantly changing and improving, and it will continue to do so. We will see steady improvements in the quality of our imaging technology, along with more widespread use. In addition, we will see the development of more advanced techniques.

Already, helical CT and some forms of magnetic resonance angiography are providing us with the ability to "see" certain things in new ways and from new perspectives. They offer three-dimensional images and rotate 360 degrees, allowing us to look at all sides of an injured area of the brain or an intracranial aneurysm. They also allow us to subtract parts of an image to look at isolated elements, like the arteries. As these technologies are perfected and put into wider use, we may eventually be able to replace such invasive diagnostic techniques as conventional arteriography. There is also hope that more detailed and sophisticated forms of magnetic resonance imaging, including diffusion- and perfusion-weighted MR, eventually may help guide the selection of patients for various types of acute ischemic stroke interventions at various times. These studies, which will help us tell which parts of the brain are still receiving blood, may benefit those who miss the three-hour window for intravenous thrombolytic therapy, for example. In addition, imaging techniques like positive emission tomography (PET) and other tools that enable us to visualize metabolism should provide further valuable information about the fundamental cellular and chemical transmissions in the brain, including vital information about the phases of illness. In fact, techniques that enable the study of basic metabolism, the processes that result in disease, and detailed pictures of the anatomy of living humans will prove to be crucial to our understanding of disease processes, including the processes involved in stroke.

TREATMENT

Stroke is often an endpoint in a lifetime of accumulated risk. We can take steps to control certain risk factors or stop their progression, but we can't undo all the damage that has occurred over the years. For that reason, it may take years before the advances in and focus on stroke prevention begin radically to change the stroke statistics, but advances in stroke treatment will be seen immediately. Ranging from minor changes in hospitalization procedures, to the development and improvement of medications and interventional techniques, to advances in rehabilitation, improvements in stroke treatment will mean the difference between a normal life or death and disability for many people.

Medications

The future of stroke treatment will bring the development of new medications, new drug combinations, and new delivery methods. Just look at the improvements of the last decade. Some of the medications that are now staples of ischemic stroke treatment haven't been around that long. Tissue plasminogen activator (tPA), the only drug approved by the Food and Drug Administration for the treatment of acute ischemic stroke, didn't receive that approval until 1996. The number of antiplatelet agents on the market has more than doubled in the last six to eight years. The development of new medications for stroke treatment is a given—from new thrombolytic drugs, to new combinations of drugs that offer benefits over and above their individual components. Although I don't believe any one medication is likely to be a panacea or offer a complete cure, these new drugs will likely result in modest improvements in stroke treatment—either in its actual results or in ways that make treatment more convenient for patients. For example, at Mayo, when a TIA or ischemic stroke patient needs anticoagulation, we have begun to use dalteparin, a relatively new drug related to heparin, as we are waiting for warfarin to take effect. Although this drug is similar to heparin in effectiveness, it can be given subcutaneously—as a normal shot—instead of intravenously. This enables patients to go home from the hospital up to a week earlier: we can train individuals to give themselves injections or make appointments for them at our outpatient clinic. This may seem like a minor advance, but if you're one of the many people who prefers to recuperate at home, it can make a big difference in your recovery—not to mention your hospital bill.

Other medication advances may bring more obvious results. New delivery methods for thrombolytic therapy, including delivering it directly to the clot using catheters threaded through the vascular system, and combinations of intravenous and intra-arterial delivery, could increase effectiveness, improve outcomes, and lengthen the treatment window for acute ischemic stroke. Although neuroprotective agents (medications designed to protect areas of the brain from permanent damage) have not yet been found to be effective in ischemic stroke, they may have more potential to help if given in combination with thrombolytic therapy.

Interventions

Technological improvements and advances will reach our high-tech treatment options. The studies on carotid angioplasty and refinements in endovascular techniques that will improve stroke prevention will also have an impact on stroke treatment. Likewise, new techniques and treatments will be developed.

Research indicates, for example, that lowering the body temperature may improve survival and reduce damage in some people with ischemic stroke, primarily by reducing intracranial pressure, the size of the infarct, and the amount of swelling. More study is necessary to determine whether this is indeed the case and, if so, when it should be performed. Similar research is ongoing regarding patients with subarachroid hemorrhage.

Meanwhile, researchers at a dozen companies are working to develop devices to remove the clots that cause ischemic stroke. These devices include specialized lasers, sound waves, water jets, and a catheter designed to suck out blood clots using a vacuum. All of these interventions are still in the early experimental stages, and their usefulness and safety remains to be seen. The work indicates that research into stroke treatment is advancing.

Rehabilitation

Although rehabilitation is the final step in treatment, it is by no means any less important. Rehabilitation will receive attention in the future as research continues into the way the brain is wired and how it may be rewired. Researchers are working to develop ways to stimulate the pathways that lead from affected muscles to the brain, which may encourage the use of a new area of the brain. This may ultimately be translated into new rehabilitation techniques. One such technique involves immobilizing a stroke survivor's good arm or leg so that he or she is forced to use the paralyzed arm or leg. A small study indicates that intensive use of a paralyzed arm may enable some people to rewire parts of their brain and regain control of the limb. It remains to be seen if this type of therapy will have widespread use. The National Institutes of Health is considering a multicenter clinical trial to test its effectiveness.

TOWARD A PREVENTIVE FUTURE

We are witnessing dramatic and rapid advances in stroke treatment. In the near future, we'll have access to improved diagnostics, medications, and interventions. Many of these procedures involve high technology that can be quite expensive. I would argue—and I believe that health economists would agree with me on this—that these added costs can be justified when measured against the much higher cost of rehabilitation and long-term disability.

But it's prevention that will have the biggest impact on reducing unnecessary death and suffering from stroke. Stroke prevention involves relatively lower technology, lower cost, and lifestyle choices that are very much within our control. The most efficient and cost-effective way to avoid disability and death is to intervene before stroke occurs. This will remain the case even with the high-tech advances we will see in the future. Although a high-tech laser procedure could prove lifesaving for a select group of people, low-tech preventive efforts have far wider reach. It has been estimated, for example, that a minimal reduction in the population's average blood pressure—a reduction of a mere 2 or 3 mm Hg—could prevent 10 percent of all strokes. That translates to approximately 75,000 strokes prevented each year in the United States alone. Efforts to prevent stroke risk factors such as hypertension and arteriosclerosis from ever developing would have an even more profound effect.

My hope is that as these exciting medical developments are unfolding, we will all do what we can to extend the power of knowledge over stroke; to get the word out that stroke is a medical emergency; to make the signs of an impending brain attack as widely recognized as those of heart attack; and to let people know that they can take direct action to prevent stroke. Knowledge trumps fear and denial—which is why it remains the first step down the path of a stroke-free life.

9

A Stroke Survival Manual: Questions and Answers You Need to Know

I f you or a loved one has suffered a stroke or is at risk of suffering a stroke, you probably have numerous questions—questions about finding the best doctor, working with your doctor, choosing a hospital, navigating the health care system, and dealing with stroke and its after effects. Most of my patients do. I encourage you to raise these questions with a doctor who is familiar with your personal situation. In the meantime, I've compiled a list of some of the questions I hear most often from my patients and others, along with my responses.

CHOOSING YOUR DOCTOR

Finding a doctor or specialist with whom you can work to treat or prevent stroke is crucial, but many people don't know where to start.

What Kind of Doctor Should I Consult?

The type of doctor you should consult depends upon your situation. If you have not experienced stroke symptoms and are simply interested in assessing your stroke risk and working to reduce it, your first consultation will likely be with a primary care doctor, an internist or family practitioner, who can work with you to determine whether you need to see a specialist. You can also start by seeing a neurologist familiar with cerebrovascular disease. This specialist may be better equipped to help you set up a stroke prevention program.

If you have experienced strokelike symptoms or have completed the risk assessment and found that you are at high or urgent risk of stroke, you should consult a neurologist familiar with cerebrovascular disease.

How Do I Find a Doctor?

Everyone should have a good primary care doctor. If you have experienced stroke or its warning signs or are at high risk of stroke, sooner or later you're going to need a doctor with expertise in cerebrovascular disease. But where do you find these individuals, and how do you know that they are qualified?

You should look for two basic qualities: competence and compatibility. These two qualities are both very important. The most competent doctor in the world may be of little help to you if you cannot work with him or her. Obviously, it's not in the best interest of your health to work with a doctor who isn't qualified. To find a doctor who meets both these criteria, you need to obtain some names, then do some research.

To get the names of potential doctors, particularly primary care doctors (I have more to say about specialists in a later question), ask for recommendations from doctors, nurses, and other health care providers you've worked with or know well, as well as from your family and trusted friends. This is often the best way to start, because you may be able to find out something about the doctor's practice style and personality as well as about his or her competence. If you have no one to advise you, you can also obtain names from your insurance company and doctor referral services, operated by local medical societies and hospitals and found on the Internet. Of course, there's always the phone book. Be aware that insurance companies and referral services will generally recommend only the physicians who work with them, while the phone book will list virtually all physicians in the area.

Once you have names of potential candidates, do a little research to find out if they meet your criteria. Find out about their educational background and how long they've been in practice (I offer sources of this information below). If they are specialists, find out if they're board certified in their specialty area. Doctors who are board certified in a certain field have additional training in that field, have passed a qualifying exam, and must keep current in the field. You can find out if a doctor is board certified by calling the

American Board of Medical Specialties at 1-866-ASK-ABMS or visiting its Web site, www.abms.org. You may be able to find information about the doctors you are considering from the doctors themselves, the hospitals or insurance companies with which they're associated, or the state medical board. In addition, several organizations post information on the backgrounds of member physicians on the Internet, including the American Medical Association, www.ama-assn.org, and the Association of State Medical Board Executive Directors, www.docboard.org.

If you believe you've found a doctor who fits the competence requirement, find out a little bit more about compatibility. Again, your best source of information is always firsthand—health care providers, friends, or relatives who have direct experience working with the doctor. You can also call the doctor's office and ask pertinent questions about his or her practice. Is it solo or group? How available is the doctor? Does the doctor accept your insurance? You won't truly know how compatible you are until you meet, but this and other information can give you a head start.

When Should I See a Specialist?

As I note above, you can choose a specialist to help you set up your personalized stroke prevention program. If you have actually experienced stroke or its warning signs or are at high risk of stroke, you definitely should see a doctor with expertise in cerebrovascular disease. This does not mean that you will need to see a specialist at all times for all of your care. Your primary care doctor may be able to handle some or most of your ongoing care. You should see a specialist whenever you're facing major decisions regarding diagnosis or treatment. For example, if you've experienced symptoms that could indicate transient ischemic attack, you should visit a specialist for diagnosis. In fact, you should visit a specialist for diagnosis if you exhibit any of the risk factors I list as urgent. You should also see a specialist if you've just had a stroke. And you should see a specialist if you and your primary care doctor are considering major surgical procedures or major treatments. A visit to the specialist is also in order if you've experienced a change in your neurological condition.

In some situations—right after a stroke or if you have a chronic condition that places you at high risk—you may see your specialist more often than you see your primary care doctor. In this case, he or she becomes your principal doctor, or principal care doctor. This is perfectly normal under the circumstances.

How Do I Find a Specialist?

The overall process of finding a specialist is similar to that of finding a primary care doctor. You obtain names and conduct research with the goal of finding a professional who meets two criteria: competence and compatibility. But you may need or want to take a different tack to find the names.

Often the best place to start is to ask your primary care doctor for a referral. This avenue offers two benefits: you're likely to find a specialist with whom your primary care doctor can work, and you're likely to find a specialist with whom you'll get along. As beneficial as this route can be, it's not always feasible. If you don't have a primary care doctor, don't have a suitable relationship with your primary care doctor, or you live in an area where few specialists are available, you may have to look elsewhere.

Although many people think that all neurologists treat stroke, that is not actually the case. The field has become increasingly specialized, and not all neurologists treat cerebrovascular diseases. Most major medical centers have subspecialized neurology departments in which you may find neurologists who specialize in treating cerebrovascular disease as well as neurosurgeons who specialize in performing such procedures as carotid endarterectomy or aneurysm surgery. These medical centers can be a good source of specialists' names. And, of course, there are the standard routes—insurance companies, referral services, and the phone book.

The board that certifies neurologists is the American Board of Psychiatry and Neurology. You can find out if a neurologist is certified by calling the American Board of Medical Specialties at 1-800-CERT or by visiting its Web site, www.certifieddoctor.org. An effort is under way at the American Board of Psychiatry and Neurology to certify doctors who subspecialize in cerebrovascular disease. In the near future, you may also be able to look for a doctor who is certified in vascular or stroke neurology.

WORKING WITH YOUR DOCTOR

Stroke can have long-lasting consequences, and many of the conditions that cause stroke or increase stroke risk are chronic. If you've had a stroke or are at medium or high risk, you need regular medical care. That means regular contact with your doctor. To make the most of these visits, the two of you need a good working relationship.

How Can I Develop a Good Working Relationship with My Doctor?

The key to a successful doctor-patient relationship is communication. It's what helps you make the most out of the time you have together. Since that time is often limited today, you need to know what to say and to say it succinctly and efficiently. Here's what you can do on your end to foster communication with your doctor:

Before your appointment, think about why you've scheduled it. Are you going to report symptoms, or are you going for a checkup to follow your progress? With the reason for your visit in mind, make a mental or written list of the pertinent facts. If you're going to the doctor to report symptoms, be prepared to describe the symptoms, including when and how they started, how long they lasted, and whether anything precipitated or relieved them. You might want to read about the signs and symptoms of stroke in this book or elsewhere to help you focus your comments. If you're going to report side effects of a medication, be prepared to detail what they are, when they started, and when and if they went away or worsened. If you're going for a checkup, be prepared to detail any symptoms you have experienced and to tell the doctor whether you have been taking any prescribed medications or have been following any recommended lifestyle changes. If you have questions, prioritize them, and ask the most important ones first. You should answer your doctor's questions accurately and in a straightforward manner, making sure to focus primarily on the most pertinent subject matter.

This approach helps the doctor obtain the information he or she needs in the quickest way possible. It shows your respect for the doctor, your understanding of his or her time constraints, and your interest and role in your own health care—all of which can engender a corresponding respect from the doctor.

If you're working with a doctor for the first time, you can get off on the right foot by finding out in advance how your doctor prefers to work and by complying with those preferences, whenever possible. For example, find out what records and films the doctor wants and in what format. Find out if the doctor wants them in advance or if you should bring them with you. Consider making an outline of all the major events, symptoms, treatments, diagnostic procedures, and hospitalizations you have experienced to enable your doctor to focus on the most pertinent information. You should also bring with you any medications you are taking or a list that includes the exact medical names and precise dosages of those medications. Be sure to tell the doctor of any adverse reactions you've had to any medications.

How Will I Know If the Relationship Is Working?

You will be able to help both yourself and your doctor if you realize that the doctor, like you, is human and that medicine has limits. If you take an adversarial or defensive approach, the doctor is more likely to respond in kind. If you approach the doctor with respect and friendliness, you'll likely get the same in return. Regardless of personalities, you can't expect your doctor to work miracles all the time. If your condition is chronic, your doctor cannot necessarily make it go away. He or she can work with you to help alleviate symptoms, prevent complications, and improve the quality of your life.

You play a crucial role in any form of treatment, and you have the right to be informed. If your doctor does not have enough time to answer your questions, schedule a follow-up visit or ask for time to explore the issues that are on your mind. Although it's best to do this in person, a letter or e-mail may have to suffice if time is a real factor. If your doctor will not make the time to provide you with the information you need or if there are major communication problems, consider changing doctors. The best way to have a good relationship with your doctor is to focus on the positive aspects of your relationship and to learn to work together as a team. Remember: Your doctor is on your side. He or she gets enormous satisfaction from helping you to get better.

CHOOSING A HOSPITAL FOR STROKE TREATMENT

As I mention in chapter 6, not all hospitals are equipped to diagnose and treat acute stroke. Although most hospitals have computed tomography (CT) or magnetic resonance imaging (MRI) scanners, not all have the equipment available twenty-four hours a day on an emergency basis. Not all have a radiologist on call to interpret the results of these scans. Not all have a neurologist or other doctor familiar with stroke treatment on call twenty-four hours a day. Even if a hospital has the ability to determine quickly that a person is suffering an ischemic stroke, it may not be able to offer state-of-the-art treatment. Only a small percentage of the nation's hospitals are currently equipped to deliver thrombolytic therapy. To benefit from the advances we have achieved in stroke treatment, it's not only crucial to recognize the signs and symptoms of stroke and to get help immediately, but also to get that help from the right hospital—a hospital that is equipped to diagnose stroke and handle emergency stroke treatment.

How Can I Find a Hospital That Is Equipped to Diagnose Stroke and Handle Emergency Treatment?

I recommend that you evaluate the hospitals in your area before stroke strikes so that you will know which is best equipped in the event of an emergency. This information is particularly pertinent if you or a member of your family is at high risk for stroke, but it's information from which virtually anyone can benefit.

Take some time to find out the answers to the following questions about the hospitals in your area, either from your doctor or a hospital administrator. The answers will tell you a lot about whether the hospitals in your area are prepared to treat acute stroke.

1. DO YOU HAVE AN ACUTE STROKE TEAM OR AN EXPERIENCED NEUROLOGIST, NEUROSURGEON, OR OTHER DOCTOR EXPERIENCED IN STROKE MANAGEMENT AVAILABLE AROUND THE CLOCK TO DIAGNOSE AND TREAT ACUTE STROKE?

Not all doctors are equipped to diagnose and treat acute stroke. In fact, even some neurologists and neurosurgeons lack experience in treating stroke. Both fields have become more and more specialized over the years. The best care, in general, comes from experts who are experienced in treating a particular condition—in this case, cerebrovascular disease. The need for experienced treatment is so important that the Brain Attack Coalition, a group of professional, volunteer, and government organizations dedicated to improving stroke treatment and prevention, recently put having an acute stroke team available around the clock at the top of its recommendations for the establishment of stroke centers in hospitals. The group defines an *acute stroke team* as a doctor with experience in diagnosing and treating cerebrovascular disease and at least one other health care provider who can evaluate any patient who may have suffered a stroke within fifteen minutes. The importance of time cannot be understated. Recent research indicates that even within the three-hour window, the earlier a patient receives treatment, the better his or her outcome.

2. ARE EMERGENCY ROOM PHYSICIANS TRAINED TO RAPIDLY DIAGNOSE AND TREAT ACUTE STROKE?

Because most people with acute stroke are taken directly to the emergency room, staff in that area need to be familiar with the diagnosis and treatment of stroke, to notify the acute stroke team, assist, or in cases when an acute stroke team is not available, to diagnose and treat stroke.

3. DO YOU HAVE A CT OR MR SCANNER AVAILABLE AROUND THE CLOCK FOR EMERGENCY USE?

Having imaging equipment and a qualified image interpreter available around the clock is crucial for rapid, accurate diagnosis of stroke.

4. DO YOU HAVE A NEURORADIOLOGIST OR RADIOLOGIST OR, ALTERNATIVELY, A NEUROLOGIST OR NEUROSURGEON AVAILABLE AROUND THE CLOCK TO INTERPRET BRAIN IMAGING SCANS?

Of the four professionals listed in the question, the neuroradiologist is the most qualified to interpret brain imaging scans.

5. IS YOUR LABORATORY OPEN AROUND THE CLOCK?

Rapid blood, X-ray, ECG, and echocardiography results help ensure prompt, accurate diagnosis. If the lab isn't open when you show up at the emergency room at three A.M., you're at the wrong hospital.

6. DO YOU OFFER THROMBOLYTIC THERAPY? IS YOUR STAFF EXPERIENCED AT ADMINISTERING THROMBOLYTIC THERAPY?

As I've said, not all hospitals offer this new therapy, which for some people means the difference between a life of disability and a life of ability. It's not enough to simply find a hospital that offers thrombolytic therapy; you should also seek a hospital that is experienced in delivering it. Recent data indicate that some of the hospitals that do offer the therapy aren't giving it to many of the patients who are eligible or are giving it after the three-hour window has passed. You need to find a hospital that will administer the drug to those who can benefit from it within a timely fashion. Thrombolytic therapy can worsen a stroke by causing hemorrhage or other complications and is more likely to do so if it is given at the wrong time or to the wrong person. Those most likely to know when and how to administer the drug are those who are experienced with its use.

7. DO YOU PROVIDE COORDINATED CARE FOR STROKE BEYOND THE ACUTE PHASE? DO YOU HAVE A "STROKE TEAM"?

As I explain in chapter 7, stroke treatment does not end with the acute phase. Continuing care includes treatment to prevent complications, treatment to address the underlying condition that caused the stroke, and rehabilitation. Generally, continuing stroke treatment involves an entire team of professionals, from the neurologist and primary care doctor to nurses and various therapists. It makes sense to seek a hospital that can handle both the emergency and continuing aspects of stroke treatment.

Are There Any Other Factors to Consider?

Yes. Location is also important. Once you have determined which hospital in your area is best equipped to treat acute stroke, find out how long it takes to get there. Find out if the ambulance service or services in your area serve that hospital and will take you to the hospital of your choice. You want to make sure you get to that hospital as soon as possible to ensure rapid treatment.

NAVIGATING THE HEALTH CARE ENVIRONMENT

If you or your loved one has had a stroke, you are probably dealing more closely with doctors, hospitals, your insurance company, and other members of the health care community than you have in the past. You may need services or face problems you've never needed before. Some advice may help.

What Services Are Available for People Who Have Had a Stroke?

Although stroke can change many aspects of the lives of stroke patients, numerous services are available to help them recover and cope with any remaining deficits. The most obvious of these services is rehabilitation. As I explain in chapter 7, rehabilitation is designed to help a person regain as much of his or her previous abilities as possible and to learn to adapt to any remaining deficits. It can include physical therapy, occupational therapy, speech therapy, and counseling. These services generally begin in the hospital, then continue at a rehabilitation center and/or in the patient's home.

Home health agencies can provide many of the various therapies as well as medical and nursing care right in the patient's home. They can also link you up with home health aides and personal care aides, who can help with some activities of daily living and light housekeeping. In addition, you may be able to find housekeeping services, meal services, and adult day care services in your area. For family members and caregivers, respite care (temporary care for the stroke survivor to give the caregiver a break) may be available.

Where Can I Find These Services?

Home health agencies are a primary source of home medical and nursing care and often a source of home rehabilitation therapy. These agencies can be privately owned, based in a hospital, or, like the Visiting Nurse Associations of America, nonprofit. Your doctor or other members of your rehabilitation team may be able to recommend a good home health agency in your area. In addition, these agencies are generally listed in the yellow pages of the phone book.

In addition to the services provided by home health agencies, you may be able to find housekeeping services, adult day care, or respite care services from nonprofit agencies and volunteer programs sponsored by churches and other charitable organizations, like Meals on Wheels, or you can hire a housekeeping service. Members of your rehabilitation team may be familiar with the services in your area. You can also check the blue pages of your phone book, or, if the stroke survivor is a senior citizen, contact your local area agency on aging.

How Will My Insurance Affect My Treatment?

How your insurance affects your treatment depends in large part on the type of insurance you have and the specific plan. Virtually all insurance plans recognize and cover stroke as a medical emergency, but some plans place more limitations on the care you can receive than others. A plan may, for example, dictate where you should be hospitalized and which doctors can care for you, limit the number of days you can be hospitalized, recommend outpatient rather than inpatient treatment, restrict your access to a rehabilitation center, or place a limit on the amount of rehabilitation you receive. After all, cutting health care costs is one of the goals of insurance companies and has been the driving force behind managed care. Some of the restrictions insurance companies and health plans place on care are reasonable. It doesn't make sense, for example, to offer (or pay for) rehabilitation services to a person who has no chance of benefiting from the services. But neither does it make sense to place a six-week limit on rehabilitation services for a patient who is progressing well and would benefit from continuing rehabilitation. With this in mind, you should familiarize yourself with the rules and restrictions of your health plan as well as your rights and the avenues available to you to challenge the plan if necessary.

What Avenues Are Available to Me to Challenge a Decision Made by My Health Plan?

Every health plan has procedures for filing complaints and appealing decisions. These procedures differ from plan to plan. You need to make yourself familiar with the procedures used by your plan. You also need to be aware of a few basic points that will help you in the process. For starters, begin documenting each interaction with your doctor, hospital, and health plan officials at the first sign of a problem. Keep copies of any pertinent correspondence, and ask your doctor for a copy of your medical record or ask him or her to be ready to send your record to the insurance company if necessary. You can also ask your doctor to help you by speaking to a plan representative or writing a letter to the health plan on your behalf.

The usual first step in filing a complaint or appealing a decision is to contact the plan's customer service center. All plans have these centers, and most are reachable via a toll-free phone number. Organize your thoughts before you call. When you reach a representative, explain your situation as clearly and directly as possible. In some cases, the customer service representative will be able to resolve your problem or answer your question immediately. If this is the case, ask him or her what steps he or she plans to take and when you'll hear back on your situation. If the customer service representative does not get back to you within the time he or she said or you are not satisfied with his or her response, ask to speak with a supervisor. In other cases, the customer service representative may not be able to handle your problem and may direct you to file a written complaint. You may also file a written complaint if you are unsatisfied with the response you receive from the customer service center.

A written complaint should explain your situation clearly and concisely, include documentation, for example test results or doctors' statements that back up your complaint, and indicate what action you want the plan to take. About a week after sending the letter, follow up by calling your insurance company and asking when you can expect a response. Request a written copy of the response when it's ready.

If your letter fails to obtain the results you are looking for, you will have to appeal your grievance to another level within your health plan. Most plans have several levels of appeal. As a final resort, you can contact your state insurance commissioner. Explain your complaint in writing and include copies of correspondence with your insurance plan. You can also enlist the help of your federal elected officials, and/or the Center for Patient Advocacy, a nonprofit organization dedicated to helping patients navigate the managed care system. The center can be reached at 1-800-846-7444.

What Can I Do If My Insurance Company, Health Plan, or Third-Party Payer Says I Should Leave the Hospital Before I'm Ready?

Enlist the help of your doctor as an advocate. He or she is the only one who can actually authorize your discharge, although your insurer can refuse to pay for care after a certain point. Most insurance companies and health plans have targets for how long patients with certain conditions should remain in the hospital. The targets are designed to ensure that no one stays in the hospital any longer than necessary, but some plans treat these targets as actual limits. In some cases, simply learning from your doctor that you are not medically ready to leave the hospital is all it takes for the insurance company to waive its target or limit. Your hospital, too, may be able to assist you. Some hospitals employ people to work as patient advocates and can help explain your situation to your insurer. In some instances, you may have to file a formal complaint or appeal the decision, using the steps I outline in the previous question.

ISSUES FOR THE PATIENT AND FAMILY

If you or your loved one has had a stroke, you probably wonder how the stroke will affect your life, whether the stroke survivor faces any restrictions, what services are available to help you cope, and where to find them. Although each person's situation is different, I offer some basic information below.

What Are Some of the Possible Effects of Stroke?

As I explain in more detail in chapter 2, the effects of stroke vary depending on the type, location, and severity of stroke. Some initial deficits resolve on their own or with rehabilitation. Other deficits may remain. Perhaps the most familiar deficit is paralysis, weakness, or lack of coordination of the leg, face, or arm, generally on one side of the body. These conditions, obviously, can affect a stroke survivor's mobility. Other possible physical deficits include loss of feeling and position on one side of the body, loss of awareness or forgetting objects on the opposite side of the body, lack of coordination, visual problems, and difficulty swallowing.

In addition, stroke can affect a person's ability to speak and communicate, to think and reason. It can even alter personality.

What Type of Personality Changes Are Possible, and How Can I Deal with Them?

Depending on the area of the brain that is affected by stroke, a person may experience any of a number of personality changes. He or she may, for example, become less inhibited; behave impulsively; experience a decrease in judgment, motivation, or self-control; become impatient, irritable, or apathetic; or may lose control over their emotions, laughing or crying spontaneously. Personality changes can range from subtle to extreme, and often the patient is unaware of these changes.

Family members are generally the ones who notice changes in a stroke patient's personality, and if they don't know that stroke can produce changes in personality, they are often taken aback. It's important for family members to realize that if a loved one acts indifferent or aggressive, it's likely the effect of the stroke they're perceiving, not a true change of heart. The family can then address the problem head on, bringing the changes to the attention of the patient's doctor, who may not have been aware of them, and perhaps discussing them with the patient. When the patient is not aware of the changes, a family member can let him or her know about the problem in a sensitive way.

Another thing to be aware of is that many stroke patients have a tendency to become depressed, especially if their stroke was severe or they aren't recovering well. Family members should be on the lookout for signs of depression, including a depressed mood, diminished interest in activities, weight loss or gain, changes in sleep patterns, fatigue, feelings of worthlessness, and a diminished ability to think or concentrate. You need to watch for these signs and be willing to get him or her professional help if necessary. Many stroke patients can be helped by antidepressant medication or some combination of medication and psychotherapy.

The support of family members can be critical to a stroke patient's ability to work through the stages of grief, including denial, anger, and resolution. Grief is a natural response to the losses associated with stroke, but dealing with the grief can be one of the most challenging aspects of rehabilitation.

One of my patients, Ralph, was a fifty-five-year-old workaholic with multiple atherosclerotic blockages in his intracranial arteries. The resulting ischemic stroke appeared as "stuttering" type episodes, which means they came on and then left, and then came on again. Over a period of two weeks, they came and went, each time causing deficits that would improve a little before the next episode.

Within a month, we had his medical situation under control, but Ralph was very depressed. He wasn't used to being sick, and he was coming to the realization that he would have to change his lifestyle and work style if he wanted to recover and stay healthy. In addition to being depressed, Ralph also exhibited some temporary personality changes that are not uncommon in stroke patients. He could be unexpectedly hostile, especially to family members, and he sometimes lost normal social inhibitions, to the point where he would say hurtful or angry things to people.

Ralph was very fortunate to have a family that circled around him in his time of crisis. After I explained to them that his hostility was a hopefully temporary result of his stroke, and that his depression was treatable, they were able to deal with the situation constructively rather than take his behavior personally. His three brothers each took time off from work to be with him, and together they were able to help him through a difficult life transition. They helped talk him through many of his concerns and helped him reevaluate his priorities, encouraging him to look at his situation as an opportunity for growth and change. He refocused his energies, which had previously centered around work, to himself and his family. He began to develop new activities and new friends. With his family's encouragement, he also sought professional psychiatric help, which was instrumental in his recovery. Thanks to his family's unstinting support, Ralph eventually recovered from almost all of the physical and emotional effects of his stroke.

What Types of Restrictions Will I Face as a Result of My Stroke?

You may be surprised to learn that most stroke patients face few restrictions, unless their stroke is complicated by coronary artery disease or another cardiac disorder that carries restrictions of its own.

In general, if you've had a transient ischemic attack or an ischemic stroke, we recommend that you stay clear of elective surgery of all kinds for about six weeks and, if possible, up to six months. This is because some areas of the brain may be damaged or marginally functional, and we don't want to subject them to the rigors of general anesthesia and blood pressure fluctuations that could kill off the cells in that marginally functional area.

We generally don't restrict physical activity, unless of course a heart condition or physical disability prohibits it. In fact, with physical and intellectual disability, we encourage patients to use the affected parts as much as possible as part of their rehabilitation. We simply ask that they try to avoid activities that could cause them to fall down and hurt themselves or bleed, particularly if they are on antiplatelet or anticoagulant therapy.

What Else Should I Know About Antiplatelet or Anticoagulant Therapy?

Antiplatelet and anticoagulant therapy thin the blood. This helps prevent the formation of clots, but it also makes bleeding more likely or more difficult to stop when it does occur. If your doctor prescribes antiplatelet or anticoagulant therapy, you need to take the medication exactly as directed. If you're taking warfarin (Coumadin), you also need to have regular blood tests to measure your blood's ability to clot. This determines your dosage. Various factors can affect your blood's clotting ability and the effectiveness of anticoagulants such as warfarin. For instance, vitamin K counteracts the effectiveness of warfarin, requiring higher doses; certain medications can also affect the way the drug works. A list of these medicines and foods containing vitamin K is in chapter 4.

In addition to monitoring your intake of vitamin K and your blood clotting time, you need to try to avoid activities that will cause bleeding or bruising. Avoid contact sports and other activities that convey a high injury risk. Be careful when handling sharp objects. Wear shoes or slippers to protect your feet. Don't trim your corns or calluses yourself. Wear a helmet when riding a bike or playing rough contact sports. Make sure throw rugs are not going to slide, and put nonskid rubber mats on floors. Use a soft toothbrush. And opt for an electric razor.

You should also be familiar with the signs of bleeding so that you can call your doctor at any sign of trouble. These include obvious signs: prolonged bleeding from a cut, your gums, or your nose; vomiting or coughing up blood; rectal bleeding; and unusually heavy menstrual flow. They also include less obvious signs: red or black stools, red or dark brown urine, dizziness or weakness, unexplained bruising or purple areas in the skin, diarrhea or bleeding hemorrhoids, unusually prolonged headaches, or severe stomach or back pain, swelling or pain with or without bruising.

When Will I Be Able to Go Home from the Hospital or Rehabilitation Center?

The answer to that question, of course, depends on the severity of your stroke and the type of and severity of deficits it caused. Generally speaking, you can go home when you have mastered the activities of daily living that you can master or reached the point at which you can keep working on these activities at home with adequate support. You need to have learned how to compensate for your deficits and have arranged for the medical care you need to be delivered at home and for a caregiver. Your home also must be suitable. If you now use a wheelchair, you cannot access a second-floor apartment in a building without an elevator. In this case, you may have to find another place to live. You may also have to find alternate living arrangements if you require medical care that cannot be delivered at home or if you previously lived alone and cannot find someone to help you with your care. In these cases, a variety of assisted living options are available to you.

Your rehabilitation team and, often, a social worker employed by the hospital or rehabilitation center can determine when you are ready to go and help you evaluate your home to determine whether it is suitable or whether it can be adapted to meet your needs.

What Types of Home Adaptations Can Be Made?

That depends on the home itself and your needs. Some changes are as simple as transforming the use of a room: you might, for example, have the furnishings of your second-floor bedroom moved to a room on the first floor. Other changes require construction and remodeling. If you use a wheelchair, for example, you may need to build an entrance ramp to your house or to widen your doorways. Still other changes fall in between. If you use a wheelchair or have difficulty walking, you may want to replace deep-pile carpeting, secure electrical cords, rearrange furniture, or install handrails. Consult with your rehabilitation team for changes that may be applicable to your own home.

In addition to adapting your home, you can purchase a number of objects to make activities easier. If you or your loved one has difficulty when eating, for example, you might benefit from a "rocker knife" with a built-up handle that makes it easy to cut food with a minimum of hand movement, or suction cups to place at the bottom of dishes to prevent them from sliding when you eat. Likewise, a bench placed in the shower or a handheld showerhead can make it possible for a person with poor balance to shower. And easy-on, easy-off clothing or clothing that uses Velcro can be much easier to put on. Your occupational therapist can help you locate other tools that can make life easier.

Once I'm Home, Is There Anywhere I Can Turn for Support?

There certainly is. For starters, your primary care doctor and neurologist will be available to help you deal with any major problems you may encounter and help you take steps to prevent a future stroke. Other members of your rehabilitation team may remain available after you leave the hospital or rehabilitation center. You may add new members to your team, especially if you continue to receive therapy or other treatments at home. The therapists and nurses who provide home care may not be the same ones who served on your initial rehabilitation team, but they should be familiar with the situations experienced by stroke patients and their families. Last but not least, support groups and stroke clubs are available to put you in touch with others who have experienced stroke and help you cope. Your rehabilitation team may be able to put you in touch with a group in your area; many hospitals and rehabilitation centers sponsor their own clubs. You can also find a stroke club in your area by contacting the National Stroke Association or American Stroke Association, listed in Appendix B.

Epilogue

After spending an entire book discussing disease and disability, I'd like to close with a few words about health and life.

People often ask me if I find my work discouraging. After all, they say, so many people you treat are mortally ill, or already severely disabled. But when I treat my patients, I'm always struck by the life energy within them that's resisting disease. When I visualize the inside of a clogged artery, I see a powerful force trying to circulate life-giving blood to the brain and other irreplaceable organs. I see the dynamic life force within each of us struggling to persist into the future. That's what's so amazing to me about our bodies and spirits—we are each life-driven dynamos, pushing forward to express ourselves in a dizzying variety of ways. Simply put, our bodies love life.

This life force is our great gift, and our great equalizer. Many things in life are beyond our control. But we are each entrusted with an opportunity to live to the fullest and to take full advantage of those aspects of our life that we can control. As I've detailed in this book, adopting a brain-healthy lifestyle is a life-enhancing choice we can each make.

For most of us, the greatest rewards of life are touching and being touched by others. As we grow older, we understand that our actions, and our health, don't just affect us. None of us is an island. There are so many people—our families and friends, our colleagues, our neighbors—who depend on us for guidance and inspiration. I know how many people I've relied on at different stages of my life and career, how much of what I know I've learned from teachers, mentors, patients, family, and friends.

When I think about patients and loved ones who died too soon, I'm struck by what could have been, of opportunities lost: the teachers who left students behind; the artists whose best work went unfinished; the husbands and wives who missed out on their retirement dreams; the mothers and fathers who never toasted each other at their children's weddings, never taught their grandchildren a favorite poem.

As someone who's fast approaching fifty, I'm heartened by how progress both in medical science and in our society has extended the potential for the later stages of our lives. I've talked a lot in this book about recent and imminent advances in medical science. But an even more profound evolution over the past few decades has been our society's concept of what's possible in late life.

Not very long ago, fifty-five was considered an advanced age, and sixty symbolized the end of most active careers. But today, turning fifty can be the middle of life, and a sixtieth birthday can mark the beginning of a new chapter in a lengthy chronicle of achievements and pursuits. Despite the youth-orientation of many aspects of our culture, we've come to realize that with advancing age comes the maturity, vision, and wisdom that can make dreams realities for the first time in our lives. Every day I see people in their sixties and seventies who are reinventing their lives, starting new careers or relationships, pursuing newfound interests and passions.

I hope that this book has given you a clear motivation for embracing stroke prevention, and disease prevention in general. It's all about preserving the opportunities that lie ahead of us. It's about protecting the future possibilities. And the time to start is now.

Body Mass Index

Body Mass Index (BMI) takes into account your weight and height. Use the chart below to determine your BMI. A BMI of 19 to 24 is considered a healthy weight. A BMI between 25 and 29 is considered overweight. A BMI of 30 or more is considered obese.

BMI	19	24	25	26	27	28	29	30	35	40	45
Height	Weight (in pounds)										
4' 10"	91	115	119	124	129	134	138	143	167	191	215
4' 11"	94	119	124	128	133	138	143	148	173	198	222
5' 0"	97	123	128	133	138	143	148	153	179	204	230
5' 1"	100	127	132	137	143	148	153	158	185	211	238
5' 2"	104	131	136	142	147	153	158	164	191	218	246
5' 3"	107	135	141	146	152	158	163	169	197	225	254
5' 4"	110	140	145	151	157	163	169	174	204	232	262
5' 5"	114	144	150	156	162	168	174	180	210	240	270
5' 6"	118	148	155	161	167	173	179	186	216	247	278
5' 7"	121	153	159	166	172	178	185	191	223	255	287
5' 8"	125	158	164	171	177	184	190	197	230	262	295
5' 9"	128	162	169	176	182	189	196	203	236	270	304
5' 10"	132	167	174	181	188	195	202	209	243	278	313
5' 11"	136	172	179	186	193	200	208	215	250	286	322
6' 0"	140	177	184	191	199	206	213	221	258	294	331
6' 1"	144	182	189	197	204	212	219	227	265	302	340
6' 2"	148	186	194	202	210	218	225	233	272	311	350
6' 3"	152	192	200	208	216	224	232	240	279	319	359
6' 4"	156	197	205	213	221	230	238	246	287	328	369

Recommended Resources

Agency for Healthcare Research and Quality
(Formerly the Agency for Healthcare Policy and Research)
2101 E. Jefferson St., Suite 600
Rockville, MD 20852
301-594-1360
Agency of the U.S. Department of Health and Human Services that offers information on assessing the quality of health plans.

American Academy of Neurology
1080 Montreal Ave.
St. Paul, MN 55116
651-695-1940
www.aan.com
Professional society for neurologists; provides patient information on neurological conditions; Web site helps patients locate neurologists in their area.

American Heart Association
7272 Greenville Ave.
Dallas, TX 75231
800-553-6421
888-4-STROKE
www.americanheart.org
Provides information on heart disease, hypertension, and stroke.

American Stroke Association
7272 Greenville Ave.
Dallas, Texas 75231
888-4-STROKE
800-553-6321
Provides information on stroke and stroke support groups; publishes Stroke Connection *magazine; sponsors a "warmline."*

Center for Patient Advocacy
1350 Beverly Road, Suite 108
McLean, VA 22101
800-846-7444
www.patientadvocacy.org
Helps patients navigate the health care system and assists with problems.

Harvard's Whole Brain Atlas
www.med.harvard.edu/AANLIB/home.html
Web site that offers pictures of the brain and depicts the effects of stroke.

Healthfinder
www.healthfinder.gov
Web site of the U.S. Department of Health and Human Services; provides information on various conditions, offers links to databases, libraries, and on-line journals.

Mayo Clinic Division of Cerebrovascular Diseases
Mayo Clinic
Division of Cerebrovascular Diseases
200 S.W. First Street
Rochester, MN 55905
507-284-9735
507-284-4270 (fax)
www.mayo.edu/cerebro/education/stroke.html
Provides information on stroke treatment and prevention.
www.mayoclinic.com
Provides general medical information.

National Aphasia Foundation
P.O. Box 1887
Murray Hill Station
New York, NY 10156-0611
800-922-4622
www.aphasia.org
Provides information about aphasia; publishes newsletter.

National Family Caregivers Association
10400 Connecticut Ave. #500
Kensington, MD 20895-3944
800-896-3650
www.nfcacares.org
Provides information, education, and support to family caregivers.

National Heart Lung & Blood Institute
NHLBI Information
P.O. Box 30105
Bethesda, MD 20824-0105
301-592-8573
www.nhlbi.nih.gov
Federal government organization that conducts research and provides information about the causes, prevention, diagnosis, and treatment of diseases of the heart, blood vessels, blood, and lungs.

National Institute of Neurological Disorders and Stroke
Neurological Institute
P.O. Box 5801
Bethesda, MD 20824
800-352-9424
www.ninds.nih.gov
Federal government organization that conducts research and provides information about the causes, prevention, diagnosis, and treatment of neurological disorders, including stroke.

National Stroke Association
9707 E. Easter Lane
Englewood, CO 80112-3747
303-649-9299
800-STROKES (787-6537)
www.stroke.org
Provides information on stroke, including information for stroke survivors, care-givers, and family members; offers referrals to stroke support groups; provides information about products and services (including adaptive equipment and clothing) useful to stroke survivors and their families.

Neuroguide
www.neuroguide.com
Searchable index of neuroscience resources available on the Internet.

Suggested Reading

Benson, Herbert. *The Relaxation Response,* updated and expanded version. New York: Avon Books, 2000.

Bodger, Carole. *Smart Guide to Relieving Stress.* New York: John Wiley & Sons, 1999.

Callan, Ginny. *Horn of the Moon Cookbook.* New York: HarperCollins, 1987.

Caplan, Louis R., Mark L. Dyken, and J. Donald Easton. *American Heart Association Family Guide to Stroke Treatment, Recovery, and Prevention.* New York: Random House, 1994.

Covey, Stephen R. *The Seven Habits of Highly Effective People.* New York: Simon & Schuster, 1989.

Criscuolo, Claire. *Claire's Italian Feast.* New York: Penguin, 1998.

Cunningham, J. Barton, Ph.D. *The Stress Management Sourcebook: Everything You Need to Know.* Los Angeles: NTC/Contemporary Publishing Group, 1998.

Donnan, Geoffrey, and Carol Burton. *After a Stroke: A Support Book for Patients, Caregivers, Families and Friends.* Berkeley, Calif.: North Atlantic Books, 1992.

Dreher, Diane. *The Tao of Inner Peace.* New York: HarperPerennial, 1991.

Einstein, Albert. *The World As I See It.* New York: Carol Publishing Group, 1995.

Elliot, Rose. *The Complete Vegetarian Cuisine.* New York: Random House, 1996.

———. *Rose Elliot's Vegetarian Fast Food.* New York: Random House, 1996.

Fontana, David. *Learn to Meditate: A Practical Guide to Self-Discovery and Fulfillment.* San Francisco: Chronicle Books, 1999.

Gawain, Shakti. *Creative Visualization,* revised and updated. New York: New World Library, 1995.

Gee, Judee. *Intuition: Awakening Your Inner Guide.* York Beach, Maine: Samuel Weiser, 1999.

Gelles, Carol. *1,000 Vegetarian Recipes.* Hungry Minds, 1996.

George, Mike. *Learn to Relax: A Practical Guide to Easing Tension and Conquering Stress.* San Francisco: Chronicle Books, 1998.

Gersh, Bernard J., M.D., ed. *The Mayo Clinic Heart Book,* Second Edition. New York: William Morrow, 2000.

Grogan, Bryanna Clark. *The Almost No-Fat Cookbook.* Book Pub. Co., 1994.

Hagen, Philip T., ed. *Mayo Health Quest Guide to Self Care,* Rochester, Minn.: Mayo Foundation, 1997.

Harman, Willis, and Howard Rheingold. *Higher Creativity: Liberating the Unconscious for Breakthrough Insights.* Los Angeles: Jeremy P. Tarcher, 1984.

Hayward, Susan. *A Guide for the Advanced Soul: A Book of Insight.* Hayward Books, 2000.

Hensrud, Donald, ed. *The Mayo Clinic Williams Sonoma Cookbook.* New York: Time-Life Books (Weldon Owen Inc., San Francisco), 1998.

Katzen, Mollie. *The New Moosewood Cookbook.* Berkeley, Calif.: Ten Speed Press, 2000.

Larson, David E., ed. *Mayo Clinic Family Health Book,* 2d ed. New York: William Morrow, 1996.

Lehrman, Fredric. *The Sacred Landscape.* Berkeley, Calif.: Celestial Arts Publishing, 1988.

Madison, Deborah, and Edward Espe Brown. *The Greens Cookbook.* New York: Bantam, 1987.

Migliaccio, Janice. *Follow Your Heart's Vegetarian Soup Cookbook.* Santa Barbara, Calif.: Woodbridge Press, 1983.

Milne, Courtney. *The Sacred Earth.* Saskatoon, Saskatchewan: Prairie Books, 1991.

Ornish, Dean. *Love and Survival.* New York: HarperCollins, 1998.

————. *Reversing Heart Disease.* New York: Ballantine Books, 1990.

————, et al. *Everyday Cooking with Dr. Dean Ornish.* New York: Harper-Collins, 1997.

Roche, Lorin. *Meditation Made Easy.* New York: Harper San Francisco, 1998.

U.S. Department of Health and Human Services, Agency for Health Care Policy and Research. *Clinical Practice Guideline No. 16, Post-Stroke Rehabilitation.* AHCPR Publication No. 95-0662, May 1995.

Weil, Andrew. *Eating Well for Optimum Health.* New York: Alfred A. Knopf, 2000.

White, John, ed. *What Is Enlightenment? Exploring the Goal of the Spiritual Path.* Paragon House, 1995.

Wiebers, David O., Valery L. Feigin, and Robert D. Brown Jr. *Cerebrovascular Disease in Clinical Practice.* Boston: Little, Brown, 1997.

————. *Handbook of Stroke.* Philadelphia: Lippincott-Raven Publishers, 1997.

Wilber, Ken. *Quantum Questions: Mystical Writings of the World's Great Physicists.* New York: Random House, 1984.

D

Brain-Healthy Recipes

The recipes below are for meal plans described in chapter 5, "The Stroke-Free for Life Prevention Plan."

SHEPHERD'S PIE

SERVES 4

PREPARATION TIME: 45 MINUTES

3 TBSP. OLIVE OIL

½ MEDIUM ONION, CHOPPED

I CLOVE GARLIC, MINCED

I PACKAGE (12 OZ.) FROZEN SOY VEGETABLE CRUMBLES

I CAN LOW-SODIUM TOMATO SOUP

I CUP FRESH, FROZEN, OR CANNED GREEN BEANS

MASHED POTATOES

Preheat oven to 425 degrees. Heat olive oil in large skillet over medium heat. Add onion, then garlic, and cook 5–7 minutes. Add soy vegetable crumbles, tomato soup, and beans, and blend. Pour mixture into deep pie dish or shallow casserole dish. Spread mashed potatoes over top.

Bake in oven for 20–30 minutes.

OVEN ROASTED VEGETABLES WITH PASTA

SERVES 4

PREPARATION TIME: 90 MINUTES

> I YELLOW OR GREEN PEPPER, CHOPPED
>
> I RED SWEET PEPPER, CHOPPED
>
> 2 EGGPLANTS, CHOPPED
>
> I LARGE ONION, CHOPPED
>
> $\frac{1}{3}$ CUP OLIVE OIL
>
> RED PEPPER FLAKES (OPTIONAL)
>
> I POUND SHORT (TUBE, RIGATONI, OR YOUR FAVORITE
> SHORT STYLE) PASTA
>
> JUICE OF $\frac{1}{2}$ LEMON
>
> PARMESAN CHEESE (OPTIONAL)

Place chopped peppers on large cookie sheet, add chopped eggplant and onion. Pour olive oil evenly over vegetables. Sprinkle with red pepper flakes if desired. Stir slightly to mix. Place in 350 degree oven for 15 minutes. Remove from oven, mix vegetables, and return to oven. Repeat, mixing every 15 minutes, for 60 to 90 minutes (until nicely roasted and browned). During the last half-hour or so of roasting, bring large pot of water to boil and prepare pasta according to package directions. When vegetables are done, remove from oven, squeeze lemon juice over all, and mix. Drain pasta and mix with roasted vegetables. Sprinkle Parmesan cheese over top if desired.

GREEN BEAN DINNER MEDLEY

SERVES 4–6

PREPARATION TIME: 1½–2 HOURS

> 1½–2 POUNDS FRESH GREEN BEANS, WASHED AND CUT
>
> 2–3 SLICES FRESH ONION, CHOPPED
>
> 2–3 TBSP. IMITATION BACON BITS

2–3 CARROTS, PEELED AND CHOPPED

4–5 MEDIUM POTATOES, PEELED AND CUT INTO QUARTERS

Cover beans with water and add the 2 or 3 slices of chopped onion and imitation bacon bits. Cover and cook over medium heat until beans are partially cooked, then add carrot pieces. After another 10 minutes of cooking, add peeled potato pieces and cook another 30–40 minutes, or until potatoes are tender. One potful does it!

PORTOBELLO MUSHROOM BURGERS

SERVES 2

PREPARATION TIME: 30 MINUTES

1½ TBSP. CANOLA OR OLIVE OIL

½ CUP MINCED ONION

I LARGE GARLIC CLOVE, MINCED

3½–4 CUPS PORTOBELLO MUSHROOMS, DICED

½ CUP HERB-SEASONED BREAD CRUMBS

I EGG

FRESH BLACK PEPPER

Sauté the onion and garlic in oil for 15–20 minutes, stirring frequently. Cool. Add mushrooms, bread crumbs, egg, and pepper. Mix and form into patties. Grill until heated.

BELL PEPPERS WITH SPANISH RICE

SERVES 4

PREPARATION TIME: I HOUR

4 MEDIUM-LARGE GREEN BELL PEPPERS, PARBOILED

⅓ CUP FINELY CHOPPED ONION

⅓ CUP FINELY DICED GREEN PEPPER

I–2 TBSP. OLIVE OIL OR FAT-FREE MARGARINE

1½ CUPS LONG GRAIN WHITE RICE

I PACKAGE (12-OUNCE) MORNINGSTAR FARMS OR YOUR
   FAVORITE BURGER-STYLE (VEGGIE) RECIPE CRUMBLES

2 TBSP. TOMATO PASTE

I (16-OUNCE) CAN TOMATO SAUCE

I–2 TBSP. IMITATION BACON BITS

LOW-FAT CHEDDAR CHEESE, GRATED (OPTIONAL)

In a 10-inch skillet, sauté onion and green pepper in olive oil or fat-free margarine. Cook on low heat until onion is transparent, then add rice, burger-style (veggie) recipe crumbles, tomato sauce, tomato paste, and bacon bits. Then cover and cook on low for 20 minutes or until the rice is tender. Check the skillet after 10 or 15 minutes. If it is getting too dry, add a little water, then cover and continue cooking until rice is tender.

Stuff Spanish rice mixture into green peppers, place (upright) in casserole dish, sprinkle grated cheese on top if desired, and bake in a 350-degree oven for 15–20 minutes.

POTATOES RISOTTO

SERVES 4

PREPARATION TIME: 1–1½ HOURS

To make stock:

6 CUPS WATER

1 CARROT, DICED

1 CELERY STALK WITH LEAVES, ROUGHLY CHOPPED

½ ONION COARSELY CHOPPED

BAY LEAF

2 CLOVES CHOPPED GARLIC

SEVERAL SPRIGS OF FRESH HERBS (ROSEMARY, THYME, OR
SAGE)

1 VEGETABLE BOUILLON CUBE

To make potatoes risotto:

6–7 MEDIUM-LARGE POTATOES

2 TBSP. OLIVE OIL

1 MEDIUM ONION

SAUTÉ OF WILD AND/OR OTHER FRESH MUSHROOMS
(OPTIONAL)

CHOPPED PARSLEY AS GARNISH (OPTIONAL)

PARMESAN CHEESE (OPTIONAL)

In medium saucepan, combine all ingredients to make stock, simmer 15 minutes. While stock is simmering, wash and dice potatoes (peel if they're not organic). Dice the medium onion and sauté in olive oil. When onion becomes transparent, add diced potatoes and stir for about 15 seconds before adding ½ cup of the vegetable stock. Stir potatoes frequently as broth is absorbed. When liquid is almost completely absorbed, stir potatoes, scraping any browned portions that start to stick to pan, then add another ½ cup of the broth. Continue this process, stirring often, until broth is gone and potatoes are tender, creamy, and starting to fall apart. Remove from heat. If desired, stir in a sauté of wild and/or other fresh mushrooms before serving. Garnish with chopped parsley and a sprinkling of Parmesan cheese. Serve hot.

FRESH TOMATO SAUCE OVER MASHED POTATOES

SERVES 4

PREPARATION TIME: I HOUR

3 TBSP. OLIVE OIL

½ MEDIUM YELLOW ONION, CHOPPED

I CLOVE GARLIC, MINCED

10–12 MEDIUM TOMATOES, BEST IF PEELED AND COARSELY
    CHOPPED

3 TBSP. CHOPPED PARSLEY

½ CUP CHOPPED BASIL

I BAY LEAF

2 TBSP. CHOPPED SAGE, OR I TSP. DRIED

¼ CUP WHITE WINE

A LITTLE SUGAR IF NEEDED

SALT AND PEPPER TO TASTE

Heat oil in large skillet over medium heat. Add onion and garlic, cook 5–7 minutes. Add remaining ingredients and stir, bringing to boil. Reduce heat, and continue cooking until sauce is no longer watery, about 20 minutes. Season to taste and serve over mashed potatoes.

(For low-fat mashed potatoes, boil your favorite type of potatoes in vegetable broth until tender. Drain potatoes, reserving 1 cup of the broth. Mash potatoes, add a generous dollop of low-fat sour cream, add ½ cup reserved broth and whip. Add additional broth as needed to get the consistency you like.)

SPLIT PEA SOUP

SERVES 8

PREPARATION TIME: 1½ TO 2 HOURS

- 2 QUARTS WATER
- 2 CUPS DRIED GREEN SPLIT PEAS
- 3 LARGE STALKS CELERY, CHOPPED
- 1 LARGE ONION, CHOPPED
- 1 TSP. DRIED THYME
- 2 BAY LEAVES
- 2 MEDIUM CARROTS, CUT IN ½" ROUNDS
- 2 CLOVES GARLIC, CHOPPED
- 1 TSP. DRIED BASIL
- 1 LARGE POTATO, CHOPPED
- 3 GREEN ONIONS, CHOPPED
- 2 TSP. SPIKE (A COMBINATION OF SEASONINGS AVAILABLE IN MOST FOOD STORES)
- SALT AND PEPPER TO TASTE

In large pot, add water, split peas, celery, onion, thyme, and bay leaves. Bring to boil, then reduce heat and simmer, covered, for about 30 minutes. Add carrots, garlic, and basil, then bring to another boil. Reduce heat and simmer, covered, for another 30–40 minutes. Add potato, and continue simmering another 30 minutes or so. Add green onions and seasonings to taste, then serve hot.

VEGETABLE SOUP

SERVES 8

PREPARATION TIME: ABOUT 2 HOURS (NOT INCLUDING
SOAKING TIME)

$\frac{1}{3}$ CUP DRIED WHOLE PEAS
$\frac{1}{3}$ CUP DRIED LIMA BEANS
$\frac{1}{3}$ CUP DRIED GREAT NORTHERN BEANS
$\frac{1}{3}$ CUP BARLEY

Soak the above in cold water overnight, then drain and rinse. Alternatively, place the above in a pot with 2 quarts water and bring to boil. Turn off heat and allow to sit for 30 minutes, then drain and rinse.

I LARGE ONION, CHOPPED
2 TBSP. NONFAT MARGARINE OR OLIVE OIL
2 CANS (14$\frac{1}{2}$ OZ.) TOMATOES WITH JUICES,
    DICED AND PEELED
3 TSP. SUGAR
2 QUARTS WATER
2 MEDIUM CARROTS, CUT IN $\frac{1}{2}$" ROUND
2 LARGE RUSSET POTATOES (OR 3–4 MEDIUM SIZE), CUT INTO
    $\frac{3}{4}$" PIECES
SALT AND PEPPER TO TASTE

In nonfat margarine or olive oil, sauté onion until it is soft and transparent. Add the tomatoes, sugar, water, peas, lima beans, pea beans, and barley. Bring to a boil, then reduce heat and simmer for about 1½ hours. Add the carrots and potatoes and simmer another 20–30 minutes (or until carrots and potatoes are tender). Add salt and pepper to taste, then serve.

WILD MUSHROOM GRAVY

This is a really exceptional gravy that can be served over noodles or mashed potatoes. It is especially wonderful for holiday feasts.

SERVES 6

PREPARATION TIME: MUSHROOM STOCK, 90 MINUTES;
GRAVY, 15 MINUTES

To make mushroom stock:

1 ONION, CHOPPED

2 RIBS CELERY, CHOPPED

2 CLOVES GARLIC, MINCED

1 TSP. OLIVE OIL

¾ LB. WHITE MUSHROOMS, COARSELY CHOPPED

7 CUPS WATER

1 CUP DRY WHITE WINE OR WATER

2 OZ. DRIED WILD MUSHROOMS (OYSTER, OR OTHER WILD
    MUSHROOM OF YOUR CHOICE)

8 SPRIGS PARSLEY

1 TSP. DRIED SAGE LEAVES (OR FOUR LEAVES OF FRESH SAGE)

1 TSP. DRIED THYME LEAVES (OR FOUR SPRIGS OF FRESH
    THYME)

2 TSP. BLACK PEPPERCORNS

Sauté onion, celery, and garlic in oil for 5–7 minutes. Add white mushrooms and cook 3 or 4 minutes. Add remaining ingredients and heat to boiling; reduce heat and simmer, covered, for about 1 hour. Strain stock, season with salt and pepper.

To make gravy:

3 TBSP. MARGARINE

6 TBSP. FLOUR

6 CUPS MUSHROOM STOCK (ABOVE)

2 TBSP. TOMATO SAUCE

CORNSTARCH FOR ADDITIONAL THICKENING (OPTIONAL)

Melt margarine and add flour, cooking over low heat for 1–2 minutes, whisking constantly. Gradually add mushroom stock, whisking to keep it smooth. Stir in tomato sauce, season with salt and pepper. If thicker gravy is desired, add a little cornstarch to half a cup of mushroom stock, then whisk into gravy.

Index